Next

The Coming Era in Medicine

Next

The Coming Era in Medicine

Holcomb B. Noble

General Editor

Little, Brown and Company   Boston   Toronto

FIRST EDITION

Library of Congress Cataloging-in-Publication Data

Next, the coming era in medicine.

1. Medicine.   2. Medicine — Research.   I. Noble, Holcomb B.
II. Title: Coming era in medicine.
[DNLM: 1. Medicine — trends — popular works.
WB 130 N567]
R852.N48   1987   610   87-22808
ISBN 0-316-61132-8
ISBN 0-316-61134-4 (pbk.)

FG

*Published simultaneously in Canada
by Little, Brown & Company (Canada) Limited*

PRINTED IN THE UNITED STATES OF AMERICA

Contents

Acknowledgement

Grateful acknowledgement is made to Cory Dean, assistant science editor of *The New York Times*, and Brenda Nicholson, administrative assistant in the newspaper's Science Department, without whose editorial skill and assistance the "Next" series could never have been completed. Similar gratitude is extended to Sam Summerlin, president of The New York Times Syndication Sales Corporation, whose energy and enthusiasm made it all happen.

Introduction

By Holcomb B. Noble

Holcomb B. Noble is Science and Health Editor of The New York Times Magazines.

Dr. J. Michael Bishop stepped to the podium in November 1982, at a gathering of the most prestigious scientists in America. He is a pleasant-looking man, not imposing, not intimidating. In fact, he looks a bit too young, really, to know what he's talking about. But as he began speaking, you got the feeling that, here before you, someone was striking a great heralding bell that was resounding through the halls of medical science. Michael Bishop will probably win the Nobel Prize, though that is not why the bell was ringing. It sounded, instead, because of the words he spoke and because of the tone he used. His voice was grave; it had an urgency about it; he was disturbed, upset, moved by the facts he laid out. But, at the same time, there was a powerful and persistent overtone of optimism and excitement:

"One person out of every four in this room will develop cancer," he said, pausing. "These are tragic dimensions." But then he said that these dimensions are beginning to seem no larger than the intellectual challenge they present. Every minute, 10 million cells divide in our bodies. The divisions usually occur in the right place, at the right time, in the right way — governed by mechanisms we don't understand. When the mechanisms fail, cancer develops. Why? How?

Bishop and many others have devoted their lives to finding the answers. For years such information and goals had seemed far remote. But, then, earlier in this century, things began to change. Early one morning in 1925, Robin Fahraeus became the first person to witness a biological molecule sediment in a gravitational field. To some, this might seem an abstruse event. Fahraeus thought otherwise. He roused his colleague, The Svedberg, from sleep with a phone call and a memorable message: "The," he said, "I have seen a dawn." As Fahraeus watched through a tiny glass window, the blood protein he had chosen for his experiments was moving down a centrifuge tube, leaving behind a yellow glow. Fahraeus knew from the glow that soon the structure of living matter would be laid out in fine detail, for all to see and understand. Molecular biology — the crowning glory of the twentieth-century life sciences — had been born.

Now, because of Fahraeus, because of Francis Crick and James Watson, because of Michael Bishop and Harold Varmus and Hidesaburo Hanafusa and Robert Weinberg and many other contemporary scientists, important medical events are coming thick and fast.

"A new dawn may now be upon us" is the way Michael Bishop put it.

Indeed, it is. What is really upon us is the culmination of the greatest revolution in the history of medical and biological science, and it will inevitably bring about more and more profound changes as this century runs out and the next unfolds. Optimism about the outcome of various medical battles against disease, optimism among Bishop and his colleagues in the health sciences of the world has never been higher. Modern medicine is now holding out greater promise of curing illness of many kinds, with many different treatments and technologies, in many parts of the world, in ways once inconceivable.

Perhaps the single most important element in the current

medical revolution and the current optimism is the double helix — the answer to the chemical structure of the inherited traits of all living things, the blueprints by which living organisms are constructed. Ever since Fahraeus woke up Svedberg in the middle of the night, scientists have known that, if they could learn the nature of this blueprint — if they could determine the structure of an organism's genetic material, its deoxyribonucleic acid, its DNA — then they would have made enormous strides toward conquering all disease. If cells were reproducing improperly and causing illness, and one knew how and why, then couldn't one stop the process and correct the problem?

In April 1983, molecular scientists from around the world gathered in Cambridge, England, to celebrate the great discovery of DNA structure thirty years earlier. The Nobel prize was waiting for Crick and Watson in the early 1950s — or a chief competitor, Linus Pauling — and they knew it. In 1953, Crick and Watson determined — as the culmination of hours of their own work as well as that of many others — that DNA forms two long, if tiny, strands wrapped around each other like the railings of a winding staircase. And this double helix contains within it specific, crucially important, arrangements that constitute genes. In the thirty years that have followed, important biological discoveries have cascaded forth, one after the other, as scientists have begun to learn about these strands of genetic information, to manipulate them, engineer them, in a variety of ways, from cloning foreign genes into embryonic mice, to transferring defective human genes into animals and then correcting the defect, to synthesizing human hormones.

The progress that has been made toward understanding the genetic factors implicated in cancer has been particularly rapid. Whereas cancer is often considered a hundred or more different diseases, research in the early 1980s has begun to suggest that most or all forms of cancer may result from a small number of genetic events that cause cells to grow out of control. Once scientists understand that phenomenon at a molecular level, there is a distinct possibility, though by no means a certainty, that they can devise ways to block it, thus preventing the development of cancer or curing it once it is detected. A leading British scientific journal,

Nature, predicted that the 1980s may be the decade when the basic genesis of cancer, its cause and origin in the body, is finally understood. Citing the richness of recent research findings as evidence, the journal said that, "for the first time, there is a chance of getting to the bottom of the phenomenon of cancer." Knowing the genesis of cancer and curing it are of course two different things. At this point, no one should confidently expect that a cure will definitely be found. But, said *Nature*, "There is a chance." Indeed, Dr. Lewis Thomas, chancellor of the Memorial Sloan-Kettering Cancer Center in New York, looks for the end of cancer before the turn of the century: "It could begin to fall into place at almost any time, starting next year or even next week, depending on the intensity, quality and luck of basic research." And Vincent T. DeVita, Jr., director of the National Cancer Institute, a federal agency, said, "If anybody had said five or ten years ago that by the year 2000 we may not have cancer, he would have been wrapped in a white jacket with his hands tied behind him. But those are not outlandish statements anymore. The speed of advance has been enormous."

This book is about these rapid strides in medical research. It concerns, too, some of the twentieth-century frustrations, the great barriers that have not as yet been scaled. Much about heart disease remains a mystery, for example. There is still the belief among some specialists that cholesterol may not, in the end, be found guilty as charged in its indictment as a chief heart-attack promoter. The lack of funds for the enormous amounts of research that remain to be done in some areas is another frustration. How do you prove or disprove that dioxin or the billions of pounds of pesticides and herbicides now used throughout the world as part of the hailed Green Revolution pose or do not pose a serious health threat? One cannot feed humans dioxin to see how soon and under what circumstances they die. Voluminous correlatives are required, so that, in the absence of direct proof, a great preponderance of evidence will point one way or the other.

So, broadly speaking, the book deals with areas in which major medical achievements have been made, and areas in which major, dramatic barriers have yet to be overcome. In some cases, it approaches these achievements and barriers on an illness-by-illness basis. In other cases, the individual chapters consist of larger categories, such as immunization or organ transplants, which transcend the boundaries of a single disease but in which dramatic accomplishments have been made or are in the offing against several sicknesses, or in which significant mysteries remain.

The book begins with two chapters on cancer, one on the intense and exhaustive research being done to discover the causes of cancer and the other on the treatments that are emerging. It also takes up the medical triumphs, as well as the failures to date, in the research and treatment of mental disorders, essentially through far-reaching discoveries about the chemistry of the brain. Organ transplantations are then described — and the marvelous tricks that have been developed for turning the complex and normally efficient human immune system off so that the body will accept foreign tissue instead of killing it as the system is designed to do. This volume also recounts the battle against the number one killer in much of the world, heart disease; the refinement of old vaccines and the development of radically new ones; and a description of the magnitude of dramatic medical problems that still exist in treating diabetes, herpes, Alzheimer's disease and, especially, AIDS.

At the end the book returns to the subject with which it began: genetics. The final chapter is on genes and the increasing understanding of their dominant importance in both causing and curing disease and on learning how to correct those genes when they malfunction. As Michael Bishop told his fellow scientists: "The enemy has been found — it is part of us — and we have begun to understand its lines of attack." Where the new genetic discoveries will take us is impossible for anyone to know. That they will succeed in the attempts to overwhelm human illness to a far greater degree than anyone could have possibly dreamed seems assured.

Next

The Coming Era in Medicine

Chapter One

The Crucial Search
for the Origins of Cancer

By Harold M. Schmeck, Jr.

Harold M. Schmeck, Jr., the author of The Semiartificial Man *and* Immunology: The Many-Edged Sword, *writes on the biological sciences for* The New York Times.

On a Saturday morning in May 1983, Dr. Russell Doolittle, of the University of California at San Diego, was at home, sitting at a computer terminal, adding another set of facts to a catalogue he had been compiling for five years. Dr. Doolittle is an expert on protein structure and evolution. Every time a new report is published on the chemical structure of a protein, or of the gene that is the blueprint for it, he puts the data in the computer. Differences in the structures of similar substances made by different species — man and mouse, for example — can reveal something of the evolutionary distance between the two species. This kind of analysis is a powerful tool for studying evolution. It has become possible only with the advent of gene-splicing and scientists' ability to read the messages of the genes.

On this Saturday morning, Dr. Doolittle was feeding the computer new data on a blood substance called platelet-derived growth factor. It is a protein that seems to play a role in the clotting of blood to heal wounds. Scientists have been studying it for at least a decade, but only recently has it been possible to decode the exact chemical message of its gene. That was the genetic message Dr. Doolittle was putting into his computer catalogue.

When the computer digested the information, it compared the new gene sequence with others already in the catalogue and found a remarkable similarity in structure between the gene for platelet-derived growth factor and that of one of the recently discovered cancer genes. That showed clearly that the two genes must be closely related and the protein products of those two genes must also be related.

This was startling and important news. It was the first time one of the cancer genes had been linked to a normal gene that had a known function in the human body. It was information of a kind that scientists had been seeking for several years.

Cancer genes, known to scientists as oncogenes, were, and still are, big news in cancer research. The fact that they existed was discovered only a few years ago, and the discovery caused great excitement among scientists.

It has been known for many years that cancer is a matter of disordered growth of cells. Although there are many different kinds of cancer and seemingly many different causes, all the forms of cancer seem to stem from a loss of normal control of the growth process. Malignant cells stop behaving as law-abiding citizens of the huge community of different cell types that make up the human body. Instead, they become anarchists, violating the body's rules, growing invasively without discipline at the expense of their neighbors.

Such behavior has always suggested that the fundamental fault must lie at the cells' most basic regulatory level, and that means the genes. That was why the discovery of cancer genes several years ago seemed to be a profoundly hopeful advance. If the genes responsible for cancer were discovered at last, scientists might hope, through studying them, to understand at last the common mechanisms that underlie all of the many forms of cancer. To some optimistic cancer experts it seemed that the fundamental riddle of cancer might now be solved at last.

But, in fact, the discovery of the oncogenes immediately raised a whole forest of new questions. Clearly they existed, but why did they exist? Where did they come from? What, exactly, did they do?

For one oncogene, at least, Dr. Doolittle's fortuitous discovery gave a strong hint on that last question. As its name indicates, platelet-derived growth factor is believed to be involved in the regulation of cell growth. If an oncogene was the blueprint for an abnormal version of that substance, might it not cause uncontrolled growth? It was this hint that caused the excitement among scientists. It appeared that the first link had been found between a cancer gene and a normal gene of known function in the human body. Furthermore, that link hinted that the oncogene did just what one might have expected it to do — affect a normal process of cell growth. The discovery impelled cancer gene researchers on an even more urgent search for the normal counterparts of other oncogenes.

These so-called cancer genes had been found originally through their ability to transform to a cancerous state cells of a particular type that are grown in laboratories for research purposes. These standard tissue culture cells are called NIH 3T3 cells. They are not cancer cells, but when certain genes from human or animal cancers are put into the cultures, the NIH 3T3 cells are transformed into a cancerlike state. They lose discipline, as cancer cells do. Instead of growing in flat sheets only one cell deep, the way normal cells grow in the laboratory, they pile up one on top of another and grow like cancer.

Genes from normal cells do not cause this malignant transformation in growths of the NIH 3T3 cells.

The first known oncogenes were found almost simultaneously by scientists in several laboratories: those of Dr. Robert A. Weinberg at the Massachusetts Institute of Technology; Dr. Geoffrey M. Cooper at the Dana-Farber Cancer Institute and Harvard Medical School; and Dr. Michael Wigler at the Cold Spring Harbor Laboratory on Long Island. In quick succession these ominous but interesting genes were found in an impressively wide variety of human cancer cells. Among them were cancers of bladder, colon, lung, and breast — some of the most important human cancers.

It began to look as if these genes might be a crucial factor in the whole complex process of cancer, and the available evidence suggested strongly that only a few dozen such genes existed at the most. Optimists speculated that these few might be responsible for the origins of all cancers and that the understanding of oncogenes might lead to one of the most important long-term goals of medical research — understanding of the ultimate nature of cancer.

One of the things that made this idea seem particularly hopeful was a different realm of cancer research that had been flourishing for many years. This was the study of viruses that cause cancers in animals. It had its origins almost a century ago when, in 1908, two Danish veterinarians, V. Ellerman and O. Bang, demonstrated that a carefully filtered and cell-free extract of blood from a chicken suffering from a form of leukemia could transmit the disease to other chickens. The fact that transmission of the disease could be accomplished by such a cell-free extract was taken as proof that the cause was a virus. In those days, before the invention of the electron microscope, little was known about viruses beyond the fact that they did cause some diseases and that, whatever they were, they were so small that they passed through filters that held back bacteria and all other microbes known to cause infectious diseases. For this reason they were originally called filterable viruses.

Historians of cancer research say the experiments of Ellerman and Bang linked cancer to a virus for the first time. Another major step in cancer virus research was taken three years later by Dr. Francis Peyton Rous of the Rockefeller Institute for Medical Research in New York, now the Rockefeller University. He did similar experiments with chickens, successfully transmitting a different kind of cancer, sarcoma, from one chick to another. Dr. Rous, who later received a Nobel prize for his research, added an important concept by showing that the cell-free extracts always produced the same kind of cancer in the chickens. From that observation, he reasoned that the transmissible agent that was causing the cancers must carry specific genetic information. For decades these highly important discoveries were ignored by most cancer research workers. The idea that viruses could cause cancer was widely viewed with contempt.

But another major advance in proving that viruses are indeed related to cancer, at least in animals, was scored in 1951 when Dr. Ludwik Gross of the U.S. Veterans Administration Hospital in the Bronx discovered a virus that causes leukemia in mice. This reawakened scientists' interest in the cancer virus puzzle. In the following years research on the relationships between viruses and cancer became an increasingly active subject.

Today it is well known that viruses are really little more than packaged pieces of genetic material — packaged genes — that wander through the world of living creatures looking for cells to infect. Inside the infected cell, the virus's genetic material subverts the cell's own machinery and induces it to make copies of the virus. Only in this way can viruses reproduce. In the process, the cell that has been invaded and subverted is usually killed.

That is the common scenario for ordinary virus infections. The virus infections that cause cancer in animals seem to be different and far more subtle. Often, the invaded cell is not killed, but its life is distorted. In ways that are still far from being understood, such a cell is transformed. Its progeny become cancer cells.

Through much of the 1950s, 1960s, and the early years of the 1970s, there was a great deal of virus cancer research, most of it supported by the National Cancer Institute. Much was learned about the nature of cancer-causing viruses and the nature of cancer itself, but there remained one giant and frustrating gap. Notwithstanding all of the evidence linking viruses to various cancers of animals, no one could find clear proof that any virus was the direct cause of any human cancer. Strong circumstantial evidence was found that a virus called Epstein-Barr virus is a causative factor in Burkitt's lymphoma, a cancer most common in African children. But the virus appeared not to be the whole story. Other factors seemed to be required for the cancers to develop. Similarly, the hepatitis B virus, known to be a major cause of liver disease in much of Asia, was linked circumstantially to liver cancers because many of those who suffered from chronic liver disease caused by the virus later developed liver cancer.

But these links between viruses and human cancers did relatively little to clarify the essential puzzle: how does cancer actually begin and how does the genetic information in viruses actually contribute to malignant transformation?

In the late 1970s and early 1980s, however, the picture changed dramatically. Unexpectedly, the disparate research fields of oncogenes and cancer viruses came together.

It had been known for years that some cancer-causing viruses carried oncogenes of their own that appeared to be responsible for the disastrous transformations those viruses caused in the cells they infected.

A key discovery changed scientists' view of those virus genes. Research by Dr. J. Michael Bishop and Harold E. Varmus of the University of California at San Francisco showed to everyone's surprise that these cancer genes were not native virus genes at all. Instead, they were animal genes that had somehow been stolen from animal cells and made part of the virus's endowment.

In their native animal cells, these pirated genes presumably have important normal functions, perhaps causing certain cells to proliferate when they need to do so in the course of normal development. At other times they are presumably repressed. That is the normal situation for most of the genes in an animal or human body. Each cell contains a complete set of the genes of the whole creature, but most of the time, most of them are quiescent, turned off. Each gene is turned on only when it is needed in the specific type of cell that requires that gene's action.

The whole process of development from a single fertilized egg cell to a whole mature creature such as a human or a great blue whale is a matter of orchestrating the functioning of tens of thousands of different genes.

When it was discovered that cancer virus oncogenes were really animal genes that had been picked up and carried off by virus particles during some long-past infection, scientists seemed to have a new opening for two important realms of study. One was the study of normal differentiation and development, one of the key puzzles of modern biology. The other, also a key puzzle of research, was the nature of cancer and the early steps that start the deadly process of malignancy. For the moment, there was no thought of native cellular oncogenes because they had not yet been discovered.

The research by Dr. Bishop and Dr. Varmus suggested a way in which the virus genes might function in the cancer process. They seemed to be perfectly normal animal genes. Yet some of the cancer viruses that harbor those genes produce cancers in an almost frighteningly abrupt fashion. Once injected in an animal, some such viruses can produce detectable cancers within a few days and kill their victims within two weeks.

Natural cancers often take a large part of an individual's lifetime to develop. Why should the animal cancer viruses do it so quickly, particularly when it seemed that the genes that did the job were nothing but normal genes of animal cells?

The highly active cancer viruses seemed to bypass the early steps by which malignancy starts.

The scientists working with these puzzling viruses could see a possible explanation. Perhaps, when a virus infection brought the oncogene back into the animal's cells, it brought in multiple copies. The extra dosage might be the source of malignant action. Or, as an alternative, perhaps the virus brought the gene to a place in the animal's genetic machinery where it did not normally go and could not reside without turning on the chaos of cancer.

The puzzle of cancer was still unsolved, but scientists had found something for which they always search; an opening in the blank wall of the unknown, a new set of facts against which hypotheses might be tested.

"We have learned an immensely important fact," said Dr. Bishop in a lecture to a group of his scientific peers. That fact was that one gene, by means of a single protein product, could induce the entire set of circumstances that make a cell cancerous.

"Know that protein, and how it acts, and you will have your fingertips on the events that generate a neoplastic [cancerous] cell."

Dr. Ray L. Erickson of the University of Colorado had identified the protein produced by the cancer gene of one of the most intensely studied cancer viruses, the Rous sarcoma virus, discovered by Dr. Francis Peyton Rous a half century before.

In their related studies of the same virus and its cancer gene, Dr. Bishop and his colleagues in California found a virtually identical gene in every vertebrate species they studied, including the human. In each case studied, the gene governed the production of an enzyme indistinguishable from the enzyme that was the natural product of the cancer virus gene.

The identity of this enzyme was particularly interesting to cancer scientists because it proved to be something called a kinase, an enzyme that has the function of adding a phosphorus atom to one of the building blocks of all proteins. This transfer of the phosphorus atom is a process called phosphorylation. It is known to have manifold important effects on living tissues and is of great scientific interest.

At just about that point in the story of modern cancer research the native human and animal oncogenes were discovered and virtually within months it was also discovered that many, probably all, of these newfound cancer genes were identical to one or another of the virus oncogenes that had been under intense study for years.

The discovery came bit by bit from several laboratories. For example, Dr. Robert A. Weinberg's group at M.I.T. reported that one of the virus genes and the human oncogenes linked to bladder cancer were virtually identical. Dr. Geoffrey M. Cooper's group at the Dana-Farber Cancer Institute and that of Dr. Mariano Barbacid, of the National Cancer Institute, also found examples of similarities so close that they probably indicated identity between virus and human or animal oncogenes.

In remarkably short order it became a matter of generally accepted scientific fact that the oncogenes, whether of viruses or human cancer cells, were the same. There were two dozen or more of them and they seemed about to give scientists a highly illuminating new view of the cancer process.

The discovery that oncogenes were really one subject was hailed by cancer research workers as a great advance. Among other things it meant that all of the decades-long research on cancer viruses and their genes could now be applied directly to understanding human cancer.

"That is a most remarkable and exciting thing," Dr. Cooper said at the time. "Ultimately one hopes to really understand the mechanisms. The hope, of course, is that understanding the detailed mechanism will suggest new approaches to prevention, diagnosis, and therapy that were not possible before."

In most areas of scientific research, advances like the discovery of oncogenes come only rarely and are commonly followed by long periods in which the details and implications of the discovery are explored in detail, but without much in the way of new dramatic discoveries.

The pattern of recent cancer research has been far different and much more rapid in its progress. For a time, new discoveries concerning the oncogenes seemed to come continually, each one adding something new and exciting to human insights into the nature of cancer. In recent years, the pace may have slowed somewhat, but the excitement still remains.

Late in 1986, scientists in Boston discovered an oncogene of an entirely different kind — an antioncogene. The research was a collaboration among scientists of M.I.T., the Whitehead Institute, and Harvard's teaching institutions: Massachusetts General Hospital, the Dana-Farber Cancer Institute, and Boston Children's Hospital.

Studying retinoblastoma, a serious childhood cancer of the eye, the scientists found the gene caused the disease by default when its influence was totally lacking. Normally, a person has two copies of the gene. In the body's normal complex system of checks and balances, the genes are believed to have a restraining influence on growth. Retinoblastoma develops when both copies are lost or inactivated.

That such antioncogenes should exist was predicted more than a decade ago. The discovery of the first example added a new dimension to the studies of oncogenes. In recent years, scientists have learned a great deal about the biology of cancer from study of oncogenes. But early hopes that these aberrant genes might be the key to solving the whole riddle of cancer have not been fulfilled.

There is still much debate as to their role. They have raised at least as many questions as they have answered.

But, today, oncogenes are a major field of cancer research, promising to help clarify important concepts of normal as well as abnormal growth.

The new research is intimately intertwined with a revolution in biology that is having profound effects on all manner of things, philosophical as well as practical. This is the revolution brought about by recombinant DNA technology, known popularly as gene-splicing.

The discovery of oncongenes was not a direct outgrowth of gene-splicing research, but the revolutionary techniques of that new field made the cancer discoveries possible and brought them to fruition far more rapidly than would otherwise have been possible; indeed far faster than cancer research had ever moved before

The pace of research quickened.

Scientists increased the list of known human oncogenes, identified new significance in the breakage and rearrangement of chromosomes as this relates to cancer, and began to see the likely functions of cancer genes' normal counterparts within the body.

One of the most dramatic early discoveries was made by Dr. Weinberg's group at M.I.T. They had succeeded in growing in the laboratory one of the most studied cancer genes and also its normal counterpart. The obvious questions arose: What were the differences between the two genes? How much of a disparity did it take to spell the difference between cancer and normalcy?

Painstakingly, the scientists compared the entire sequences of DNA subunits in the two forms of the gene. Altogether, each gene was made up of approximately 6,000 such subunits, and it was clear that the normal and abnormal versions were closely similar. But just how similar were they? It was a question that had to be attacked step by step. As the scientists compared the two more and more closely, the similarity became increasingly striking. First, the experiments showed that there could not be more than a hundred or so subunits that were different, then the possible disparity was pared down to a possible dozen subunits, then even fewer.

It began to look as though the two might actually be identical.

If true, the finding would make the biological puzzle of cancer even more puzzling.

But, it turned out that the two were not identical. Out of more than 6,000 subunits in the gene, just one differed from the others. That single difference changed the coded message in the gene just enough so that it changed one amino acid in the protein chain of 190 that was the gene's product. Instead of the amino acid glycine at a particular point in the chain, the abnormal gene product had valine. Why that single change should make such a profound difference was, and still is, a complete mystery. Could it be that the riddle of cancer was based on such seeming trivialities? No one really believed that, least of all the scientists at M.I.T. They had a clue that some day would fit into the grim mosaic of the cancer process, but it was only a clue.

Cancer scientists knew that such beautiful simplicity was flying in the face of a mountain of evidence gained painfully through decades of research. Cancer was a complex, multistage process. There could be little doubt of that. It did not seem possible that a simple substitution of one amino acid among almost 200 could account for the whole process even if the change came in a particularly vital substance in a crucially important cell.

Indeed, the tide of research soon began to turn away from simplicity again. Dr. Weinberg's group in the United States and Dr. Robert F. Newbold and Robert W. Overell of the Institute of Cancer Research in Buckinghamshire, England, found that the action of one oncogene alone was not sufficient to change truly normal cells to a cancerous state. Instead, it took two, each from a different class of oncogenes.

From the start, cancer research workers had a nagging worry about the NIH 3T3 cells. They were not cancerous, but, at the same time, the way they grew in the laboratory was not quite normal either. They probably represented an in-between stage. If so, were the dramatic effects produced by introducing one oncogene really significant?

The message of the new research helped clarify this. The experiments with the NIH 3T3 cells was indeed significant, but it did not tell the whole story. Evidently those cells had advanced part of the way along the path to malignancy before the oncogene got there. The transplanted gene did the rest.

At a scientific symposium attended by many of the leaders in research on oncogenes, Dr. Philip Leder, of Harvard University, said the cancer process should probably be thought of as a cascade in which several events, each individually minor, contribute one after another. Finally, the process of transformation, developing bit by bit, reaches a stage from which there is no turning back. The progression is almost always first detected after this stage has been reached. By that time, cancer actually exists. Supporting and amplifying this concept, he described research in his laboratory in which a breed of mice had been made permanently cancer prone by transplanting into their embryonic cells a laboratory-concocted cancer gene.

In the crescendo of this rapidly advancing research, there was always the implication that if a process becomes thoroughly understood, ways might well be found for manipulating it, even turning it off. That had always been an ultimate and often-deferred hope of cancer research.

All of cancer treatment since the first beginnings of medical science have been based on a grim scorched-earth policy. One must kill or remove the cancer — by surgery or radiation — and clear enough of the surrounding territory so that no cancer cells at all will survive the attack. The advent of anticancer drugs has meant that a substantially increased number of cancers can be halted in their tracks, but the strategy is still the same. All of the drugs are killers, too, effective only because they kill more cancer cells than normal cells.

If the underlying process of cancer could be well enough understood, a whole new and far superior strategy might be possible. It might be possible to turn off the process itself — not just kill the cancer cells, but actually halt the progression by which they formed. Experiments have shown that the process of transformation impelled by an oncogene can sometimes actually be halted in cells growing in laboratory tissue cultures. The process of transformation stops and the cell culture regains its normalcy. Research is actually under way to see if such a thing could be achieved in human cancer patients. So far, this has progressed only to the stage of testing the necessary chemicals for safety. No one expects from the research an early or easy victory, but the fact that the experiments can be conceived at all is encouraging. In the past it was always beyond rational hope.

One such set of early experiments is in progress at the National Cancer Institute as the fruit of an independent but related discovery linking viruses with cancer.

Despite the existence of the Epstein-Barr virus that is linked to lymphomas in Africa, the relationship between hepatitis B virus and liver cancer in Asia, and the frequency with which certain herpes viruses and papilloma viruses are found in some cancers of the reproductive tract in the United States, no one had ever discovered a true human cancer virus.

Many of the viruses that were so much studied in animal cancers and contributed so much to the understanding of onco-genes are of a kind called retroviruses. The name comes from an unusual enzyme with which they are equipped that seems to fly in the face of a basic tenet of modern molecular biology. This enzyme was discovered in 1970 independently by two scientific teams, one led by Dr. David Baltimore of the Massachusetts Institute of Technology, the other by Dr. Howard Temin of the University of Wisconsin. The basic principle that seemed to be violated by the enzyme was sometimes called the central dogma of molecular biology. This concept was that genetic information and action in living cells always proceeded in one direction. It went from the DNA, which is the archive of hereditary information in all living things, to RNA, the stuff of the actual working blueprints of life, to the use of those blueprints by the cell in the manufacturing of the proteins that give the cell its identity and all of its functions.

The progression was always DNA to RNA to protein. Life was organized that way in all animal, plant, and microbial cells, and it seemed to be the case also in virus infections. When any virus invaded a cell, the nucleic acid in the virus's core went to work subverting the cell's genetic machinery to produce a new crop of viruses. The core was DNA in many viruses and RNA in many others, including the animal cancer viruses.

In those viruses that contain DNA, the process seemed simple enough: the cell presumably translated the DNA into RNA and this was used as the blueprint for making new virus particles. The situation with RNA viruses seemed even simpler: the invaded cell apparently took the RNA directly as the manufacturing blueprint and used it for making new viruses.

But the discovery of the enzyme, called a reverse transcriptase, showed that animal cancer viruses could actually do it differently. The enzyme activates a seemingly heretical translation. The message of RNA is translated back into DNA — hence the word reverse in the enzyme's name — and only thereafter does the process go in the normal fashion from DNA to RNA to manufacture of protein.

In addition to opening up a vast new vista of possibilities for cancer research, the retroviruses have become a key tool of gene-splicing research that is used in laboratories everywhere.

Dr. Baltimore and Dr. Temin shared a Nobel prize in 1975 for their discovery of the enzyme.

It soon became clear that many of the animal cancer viruses that had been studied so avidly over the years were retroviruses. With the help of all of the new tools of molecular biology, their nature, origin, and influence on cells were made much more clear than ever before, but they were all animal viruses. The search for a human cancer-causing retrovirus continued in unsuccessful frustration.

That changed in the early 1980s because of research by Dr. Robert C. Gallo and colleagues at the National Cancer Institute. Dr. Gallo had been involved in research on animal cancer viruses for many years. One line of his research led him to think that he had found a human cancer virus. A great deal of further research proved that to be a false trail. But he persevered in the research and, in 1980, published the first of a series of reports that did indeed identify the first human cancer-causing retrovirus. It was first shown to cause cancers of the human blood-forming system, called leukemias and lymphomas. The virus Dr. Gallo and his co-workers discovered attacked specifically a set of white cells called T-lymphocytes that are crucial to the body's immune defense system. The virus was named HTLV for the human T-cell leukemia/lymphoma virus. It was first linked to human cancers in a small region of southern Japan but is now known to exist throughout the world, although evidently it is not a major cause of cancers elsewhere.

The virus is now called HTLV-I. A second such human retrovirus, HTLV-II, was found as well, but whether it plays any significant role in human cancer is still not entirely proved. The third virus in the family, HTLV-III, has been found to be the cause of AIDS, or acquired immune deficiency syndrome, a deadly disease that attacks its victims by destroying their immune defenses. It can also attack the patient's brain, sometimes causing dementia and related neurological problems. In the United States, most of its victims are male homosexuals or drug abusers or their sexual partners. Other discoverers of the AIDS virus gave it names of their own, LAV and ARV, but an international committee recently recommended a compromise name — HIV, for human immunodeficiency virus.

Because of the growing importance and gravity of the AIDS epidemic, HIV has been studied intensively and has led scientists to greater understanding of retrovirus biology in general.

HIV is by far the most complex human retrovirus ever discovered. It has more genes than any other of its kind and a particularly complex system for getting itself reproduced in the cells it infects. But HTLV-I has mysteries of its own. For example, it is one of the retroviruses that does not have an oncogene of its own, yet indisputably it causes cancer. Knowing that it exerts its effects on the T-lymphocytes, scientists at the National Cancer Institute have already taken the first steps in research toward putting that knowledge to practical use for cancer patients: safety testing a drug that is known, from laboratory experiments, to protect T-cells from the effects produced by the virus. The scientists have stressed that it was still far too early to tell whether the drug would have any merit in the treatment of cancer. But even the idea of using it would have been impossible without the progress scientists have made in recent years in understanding the biology of cancer and the closely related field of immunology, the study of the human defenses against infection and invasion.

Study of the AIDS virus, too, has suggested many possible

drug strategies for coping with the deadly infection. The first such drug was approved for prescription use by the FDA early in 1987. Many others are under development. The AIDS research has given scientists some provocative insights into the actions of cancer-causing viruses, but those studies are largely separate and distinct from the mainstream of cancer research.

As cancer scientists have believed for decades, cancer is a derangement of some of the most basic processes of life. The new excitement in cancer research today stems to a great extent from an all-pervasive revolution in biology that has been virtually exploding during the past decade. This is the revolution in molecular biology, paced by dramatic advances in recombinant DNA technology, by some other new sophisticated scientific research techniques, and by some key related discoveries.

One of the most important of these was the discovery of the process for making a special kind of antibodies called monoclonal antibodies. The discovery by Dr. Cesar Milstein and Dr. Georges Kohler at the British Medical Research Council's laboratory of molecular biology in Cambridge won for the two scientists a Nobel prize in 1984.

Antibodies are biological guided missiles. Each type of antibody is aimed at a specific single target. The monoclonal antibodies are far more precise in this targeting than any antibodies available before. Cancer researchers have used them to great advantage in studying differences among related forms of cancer that may have differing prognoses in terms of treatment and the patient's survival. Through the use of monoclonal antibodies as probes to detect differences between cells, for example, the blood cancer leukemia has been separated into different distinguishable types. This ability to tell one leukemia from another gives doctors a much better understanding of these diseases than has ever before been possible.

This has even been translated into new ideas for treatment: use of monoclonal antibodies, armed with lethal poisons, to seek and destroy cancer cells selectively; use of antibodies designed specifically to attack a trait of a single cancer patient's diseased cells. The latter kind of experimental treatment, used in a few cases at Stanford University Medical Center, has actually produced a complete and long-lasting remission of disease in at least one fortunate patient. How long it will last is unclear, but the remission has already continued for well over a year.

The experimental use of monoclonal antibodies against cancer has increased greatly in recent years. It still remains to be seen just how important this strategy against cancer will prove to be, but it has attracted a great deal of interest among cancer specialists.

Other scientists are still trying to plumb the mysteries of oncogenes. They have found accumulating evidence that the normal counterparts of oncogene products are probably all substances important to normal cell growth and metabolism. That brings the study of cancer closer and closer to study of the greatest mystery of all biology — how the single fertilized egg cell of any creature can develop during the relatively few months of residence in the womb into a complex, whole creature with millions of different kinds of specialized cells: a mouse or an elephant or a human being.

In such research, the lines between cancer and other aspects of life can seldom be drawn very sharply. Some research teams, for example, are working hard to develop means of treating "incurable" human genetic diseases by transplanting genes that could supply the lack produced by the genetic defect that underlies the disease. This has little to do with cancer research, but the gene-therapy specialists expect to use genetically engineered retroviruses to transplant the normal genes into cells of the patient. Retroviruses were discovered and studied intensely over the years by cancer scientists. Indeed, Dr. Richard Mulligan, one of main pioneers in developing retroviruses for this new gene-therapy purpose, does his studies in a cancer research unit at the Whitehead Institute, an affiliate of M.I.T.

On the other hand, Dr. Y. W. Kan of the University of California at San Francisco, an internationally known expert on the blood disorders called the thalassemias, has been one of the first actually to send genetically defective living cells a corrective message that erases the defect. It has been done only in laboratory experiments to date and has nothing directly to do with cancer treatment, but the feat is of precisely the kind that cancer scientists would like to use against the genetic abnormalities in cancer cells.

Cancer and normal cell development are crucial subjects that are everywhere intertwined. That is what makes molecular biology so exciting today.

Any advance in understanding normal cell development offers the hope that it will shed valuable light on the processes of cancer.

Any advance in understanding cancer is more than likely to give mankind a clearer and more powerful understanding of life itself.

Chapter Two

Cancer Treatment: Slow but Steady Gains

By Philip M. Boffey

Philip M. Boffey covers science and U.S. government science policies for The New York Times.

Back in June 1982, Vincent T. DeVita, Jr., director of the U.S. National Cancer Institute, told a conference of the American Cancer Society that "the best kept secret today is that cancers, as a group, are among the most curable of chronic diseases."

In a keynote address intended to set the major theme of the conference, he asserted that "progress is evident everywhere and occurring at an ever-accelerating rate."

His speech was both surprising and encouraging to a nation long accustomed to fear cancer as the most ruthless and intractable of human diseases. Although heart disease kills far more people in many industrialized countries, cancer, with its capacity to inflict pain and disfigurement, remains "the most feared of human diseases," according to the Department of Health and Human Services.

Indeed, it was not many years ago that doctors shied away from telling cancer victims the nature of their disease, and obituaries discreetly omitted mention of the cause of death, so awful and terrifying was cancer perceived to be. Even in today's supposedly more enlightened climate, cancer victims suffer discrimination by employers and ostracism by acquaintances who consider them hopelessly impaired and diminished. As far as most people are concerned, cancer is still deemed an inescapable sentence to a lingering and painful death.

These persisting fears of cancer have obscured the fact that scientists have been making slow but steady gains in detecting and treating the disease for the past half century and have apparently increased the rate of progress in recent years. Today, in the mid-1980s, more than half of all cancer victims in the United States can expect to survive their disease for at least five years after detection, the medical definition of a "cure."

The national goal is to push that cure rate still higher. Buoyed by their recent achievements, the managers of the American cancer program in March 1984 launched a major campaign to gain eventual domination over the disease. They seek to cut cancer mortality in the United States in half by the year 2000, a truly astonishing advance if it can be achieved. Their plan calls for preventing some cancers, by reducing smoking and modifying the diet, and for curing others, chiefly by increasing the use of today's most advanced therapies but also by finding better treatments for many advanced cancers.

Beyond the official plan, which relies primarily on the application and extension of current knowledge, lies an even bolder hope — that recent advances in the molecular biology of cancer will soon lead to major breakthroughs in understanding cancer at the most fundamental level. If the mysterious mechanisms of the disease are eventually understood, most scientists believe, it should be possible to devise far better methods to detect, treat, and prevent the baffling and elusive killer.

MEASURES OF PROGRESS

A few years ago, Arthur I. Holleb, senior vice-president for medical affairs at the American Cancer Society, exultantly described the progress made against cancer in his own lifetime. The death rate for cancer of the cervix had been reduced by 70 percent, thanks to a valuable screening test followed by prompt treatment. Choriocarcinoma, a rare tumor occurring in the uterus after childbirth, once uniformly fatal, was now highly curable by drugs. Childhood leukemia, once terribly lethal, was now cured in almost half the patients. Testicular cancers, largely lethal in the past, could now be cured in most cases. And major gains had been made against Hodgkin's disease, Wilm's tumor of the kidney, and a large array of childhood tumors.

But it is a perverse fact that the cancers that are now the most "curable" are statistically among the most rare. There has been far less progress in coping with cancers of the lung, gastrointestinal tract, and breast, the three major cancer killers in the United States, and little progress on cancers that afflict the brain, stomach, and esophagus.

"Progress has been remarkable in some cancers," said Frank J. Rauscher, Jr., vice-president for research at the American Cancer Society. "In others, it is anything but remarkable, and we haven't made much progress at all."

The chief statistic used to measure progress in "curing" cancer patients is the five-year relative survival rate, the percentage of patients who are still alive five years after their disease was first diagnosed, adjusted to eliminate causes of death other than cancer. By this yardstick, the National Cancer Institute reports major gains over the past three decades. In the 1950s, the institute says, only about a third of all cancer patients survived for five years. Now more than half do, thanks to better treatments.

But some distinguished cancer analysts believe this apparent progress is partly, or perhaps even largely, a statistical mirage, caused by changes in the way cancer is detected and defined. They say that doctors have become highly skilled at detecting microscopic tumors that look like cancer but would not actually kill anyone, an artifact that makes it look as if the doctors are curing these people even though the people would not have died anyway. The critics also contend that doctors are detecting real cancers at an earlier stage in their development than before, thus virtually guaranteeing that more people will survive five years after detection.

Neither of these gains, the critics say, is due to better treatments. "There has been disappointingly little progress in curative treatment since the middle of the century," says Richard Peto, a British epidemiologist who was the author of a major study of cancer mortality for the Congressional Office of Technology Assessment. An analysis published in May 1986 by Dr. John C. Bailar III, of the Harvard School of Public Health, and Dr. Elaine M. Smith, of the University of Iowa, found "no reason for optimism about overall progress in recent years" and "no reason to think that, on the whole, cancer is becoming any less common."

But leaders of the American cancer establishment dismiss the criticism as little more than undocumented assertions. "I think it's a bunch of nonsense," says Dr. DeVita. "We're saving thousands of lives today that weren't saved twenty years ago."

All the good news and optimistic future plans emanating from leaders of the American cancer establishment must be tempered by the realization that cancer remains a tough and intractable enemy that has repeatedly frustrated the finest minds in medicine. More often than not, past declarations that cancer is about to be defeated have turned out to be premature.

In 1971, for example, when President Richard M. Nixon helped launch a national crusade against cancer — known popularly as the "war on cancer" — he declared: "The time has come in America when the same kind of concentrated effort that split the atom and took man to the moon should be turned toward conquering this dread disease. Let us make a total national commitment to achieve this goal."

Congressmen unabashedly called for victory within five years, endorsing a resolution that "it is the sense of Congress that the conquest of cancer is a national crusade to be accomplished by 1976, as an appropriate commendation of the 200th anniversary of the independence of our country."

But, alas, cancer proved far more difficult to conquer than either the atom or the moon. The nation's atomic bomb project produced a weapon within a few years, and the nation's space program reached the moon in a decade. But a decade after the war

on cancer was launched, the disease remained stubbornly uncon-
quered.

In summing up the accomplishments of that first decade, Dr.
Henry C. Pitot, chairman of the National Cancer Advisory Board,
called the 1970s "an unparalleled decade of discovery." But he
also acknowledged that progress was slower than everyone had
hoped. "Ten years ago, there were some individuals who expected
that our achievements would be even greater, hoping that by now
the means to prevent or cure all forms of cancer would be in
hand," he said in 1981. "Those who have devoted themselves to
the cancer problem are deeply disappointed that this is not the
case. Much remains to be done."

THE NATURE OF CANCER

Cancer is frightening in part because it is so ubiquitous.
Cancer is the second leading cause of death in the United States,
and it affects the vast majority of households in the country. The
American Cancer Society estimates that some 73 million Americans now living will eventually come down with cancer; that's
roughly 30 percent of the population. Over the years, the society
says, cancer will strike three out of every four families. There is
almost no one in the country who has not had a friend or relative
succumb to cancer.

What makes cancer so baffling, and thus adds to its fearsome-
ness, is that cancer is not just one disease; it is a very large group of
diseases that can afflict both humans and animals. By official
government count, there are at least 100 different kinds of cancer,
and there may well be more than 300, if fine distinctions are
made. New findings in molecular biology suggest that all cancers
may ultimately be traced to a few fundamental changes in cellular
genes. But for the present, cancer remains mystifyingly complex
and varied.

Cancer can arise in any organ or tissue of the body. The most
prevalent cancers in the United States and some other industrialized countries are cancers of the lung, the colon and rectum, and
the female breast. But cancer can also attack the prostate, the
kidney, the uterus, the urinary tract, the mouth, the pancreas, the

brain, the stomach, the esophagus, the female ovary, the male testis, the skin, and the blood or lymphatic systems, among other tissues and organs. Cancer, in short, can occur in almost any part of the body.

Cancer is clearly a group word, a generic term that describes a wide range of diseases that have different behavior patterns. Some cancers grow very slowly, some quite rapidly. Some spread throughout the body; others don't move much from their original site. Most attack older people, but some are found primarily in children.

The chief common characteristic of all cancers is their abnormal, unrestrained, uncontrolled growth. Whereas normal cells stop growing and proliferating when they bump against neighboring cells or reach a natural stop-point, cancer cells do not. They keep proliferating out of control, forming a tumor or mass that grows bigger and bigger until it compresses its neighboring cells or invades and destroys them. The English word *cancer* is derived from the Greek word *karkinos,* meaning "crab," an apt description for a disease that claws its way through defenseless body tissues.

The chief menace of cancer is that the original malignant tumor, which is bad enough in its own right, often sends out seeds of destruction to infect distant sites of the body as well. In a typical case, some cancer cells break off from the original tumor and are carried by the blood or lymphatic systems to secondary sites, or metastases, where they start new tumors that invade still more tissues and organs surrounding the new site. Once a cancer has begun to spread through the body, the odds of being able to cure it plunge sharply.

DETECTION

The earlier a cancer is detected, the better the chances of curing it. This is because early cancers are small, and thus more readily removed than bigger tumors, and early cancers have not yet metastasized to distant sites in the body, where they become extraordinarily difficult to remove.

Doctors have slowly and steadily been improving their ability to detect hidden cancers. There is no single test that can detect all cancers and, given the large and diverse number of cancers that exist, there may never be one. But there are a number of tests and procedures that can detect some cancers while they are still very small.

The best known is probably the so-called Pap smear for cervical cancer in females, which can detect cell abnormalities that are often precursors of cancer. A scraping of cells is taken from the mouth of the uterus, smeared on a laboratory slide, stained, and then examined under a microscope. A Swedish study of some 200,000 women reported in September 1984 that Pap smears cut the incidence of cervical cancer by about two-thirds in women who had at least one such smear over a ten-year period. "This study laid to rest, for once and all, the age-old question, 'Are Pap smears effective in reducing cancer of the cervix?' " said one of the researchers. "Yes, they are."

Other standard detection procedures include a physical examination, palpation of various parts of the body in search of tiny lumps, the use of lighted tubes, or sigmoidoscopes, to examine the rectum for suspicious growths, and the use of mammography, a special form of X ray, to detect tiny tumors in the female breast.

The American Cancer Society in 1983 recommended that all women aged forty and above have regular mammograms to detect breast cancer, an extension of its previous recommendation that only those over age fifty undergo the procedure. The society said that recent technical improvements had increased the detection capabilities in the dense breast tissue of young women and had lowered the radiation doses to safer levels.

These proven screening tests are now being augmented by new tests that seek to detect so-called tumor markers, or molecular and biochemical indicators that a cancer is present. In June 1984, for example, American and French doctors jointly announced that they had developed a rapid, highly sensitive screening test for liver cancer. The test uses monoclonal antibodies to seek out and detect a protein, called alpha fetoprotein, that is put into the blood by a liver cancer. Other scientists are investigating dozens of other early-detection tests, based on various proteins, enzymes, antigens, and other substances associated with one or more cancers.

Most of these techniques are not yet suitable for screening large numbers of people, but they are being used to monitor the progress of patients known to have the disease. The long-range hope is that a combination of tests might ultimately be able to screen for and detect virtually all cancers.

Thus far, the screening tests have had only limited impact on the detection of cancer. "Unfortunately, our means of detecting cancer early have not improved greatly over the past twenty to thirty years," says Frank J. Rauscher. "This is because, biochemically, cancer cells are not a lot different from normal cells. Quantitatively, there may be more enzymes in cancer patients than in normal patients. But a substance that is truly unique to cancer has not been found. That's been the problem so far."

Most cancers are still detected because an individual or doctor becomes aware of symptoms that may indicate the presence of a cancer. Indeed, the American Cancer Society repeatedly emphasizes the "seven warning signals" of cancer, ranging from unusual bleeding to difficulty in swallowing. Self-awareness is still the major screening procedure.

DIAGNOSIS

The few screening tests now available are backed up by a rapidly growing array of sophisticated medical imaging devices that are sometimes used to detect cancer but more often to locate precisely, identify, and diagnose a tumor whose existence is already suspected. In recent years, computer-aided tomography, known popularly as the CAT scan, has enabled doctors to visualize previously inaccessible structures in the body and obtain a more realistic picture of internal masses. The procedure allows much greater accuracy in determining where normal tissue ends and abnormal tumor tissue begins, thus helping to target the treatment more precisely. Ultrasound is another recent addition to diagnostic procedures; it is less expensive and less hazardous than imaging techniques that rely on radiation, but in most cases its images are also less clear.

Now even the CAT scans themselves, hailed as a diagnostic

revolution just a few years ago, may soon be superseded, in many uses, by nuclear magnetic resonance imagers. Magnetic resonance is probably safer than the CAT scan because it relies on magnetic fields rather than radiation, and it may well provide clearer images of the body's interior. A report issued in September 1984 by the Congressional Office of Technology Assessment cited the "exciting possibility," which "remains to be demonstrated," that nuclear magnetic resonance "could prove capable of detecting malignant abnormalities at a stage earlier than is currently possible." By 1987, leading medical centers around the country were using magnetic resonance imagers to diagnose cancer, and the Public Health Service was recommending that magnetic resonance be approved for use on patients enrolled in Medicare, the nation's largest medical program. Another new imaging system under intense study, known as positron emission tomography, or PET, was being used to measure metabolic processes in different parts of the body and to follow the development of tumors on an experimental basis.

Despite all the technological advances of recent years, a definitive diagnosis of cancer still requires the skill of a surgeon to obtain a small slice of tissue from the suspected tumor for analysis and the judgment of a pathologist to identify the telltale appearance of cancer cells under the microscope. Such procedures, called a biopsy, usually yield a correct diagnosis, but like any procedure involving human judgment, error is sometimes inevitable.

TREATMENTS

Cancer treatments have experienced a major leap forward over the past fifteen years and there are predictions of an even more dramatic revolution in the decades ahead.

The most important advance of the 1970s was the rapid development of chemotherapy, or drug treatments. Now, for the first time, doctors had a weapon to use against the most dangerous forms of cancer, the advanced stages of the disease in which the original tumor has already sent out its destructive seeds and started metastases elsewhere in the body. Chemotherapy provided no magic cure for the disease, but it could at least seek out the hidden tumors wherever they might lie in the body. When the right drugs were used in the right combinations, and when the drugs were skillfully applied in conjunction with surgery or radiation, the traditional means for removing localized tumors, doctors were able to exert greater control over cancer than ever before. Even so, some of the most common forms of cancer, such as cancer of the lung, remain essentially uncurable.

Now another impending revolution may offer an even more potent weapon against cancer. The conventional therapies of surgery, radiation, and chemotherapy are about to be supplemented by an emerging fourth form of treatment, using an array of biological substances that are far more specific in their action and far less toxic to the body than the existing drugs. Nobody knows yet how important the new biologicals will be, but they are one of the chief reasons for optimism and excitement in the cancer community today.

The therapeutic gains made to date are the result of occasional scientific breakthroughs that produced better forms of treatment, followed by years of trial-and-error clinical studies that slowly and inexorably refined the treatments and improved their results.

SURGERY

Surgery is the oldest treatment for cancer and the one most capable of completely curing patients, provided the disease is caught before it has started to metastasize. If a tumor is caught early enough and is in a part of the body where it can be cut out without threatening the life of the patient, a skillful surgeon can excise the cancer completely.

Cancer surgery got its start in the last century, greatly assisted by the introduction of anesthetics that freed surgery from pain and antiseptic techniques that reduced the danger of infection. Well before 1900, surgeons were cutting out tumors of the ovary, esophagus, rectum, thyroid, and breast, among other organs. During the twentieth century, further advances in surgical techniques greatly improved the results of all operations, including those for cancer. Blood transfusions controlled the shock caused by operations, and antibiotics controlled the infections that frequently killed surgical patients. In recent years, new microsurgical techniques that reduce the extent of cutting, new automatic stapling devices to connect tissues, and new intravenous feeding techniques to nourish patients after surgery have all increased the effectiveness of cancer surgery.

By 1950, surgery alone appeared to have increased the survival rates of cancer patients in the United States from near zero at the beginning of the century to about 30 percent in midcentury. The record has not improved much since then, largely because about 70 percent of the patients already have micrometastases that have spread beyond the primary site by the time the surgeon sees them.

The most important trend in recent years has been to reduce the severity of surgery while achieving the same results. Up until a decade or so ago, for example, the standard treatment for breast cancer was the "radical mastectomy," introduced by William S. Halsted in 1890, in which the entire breast and associated lymph nodes were removed, leaving the patient grossly disfigured. But over the past decade numerous studies have shown that less radical surgery, sometimes simply removing the suspicious lump, followed by radiation to kill off any remaining cancer cells in the breast and perhaps drugs to knock out cells that have spread, can produce just as good results with less trauma to the patient. A study conducted by researchers at eighty-nine institutions, under federal sponsorship, concluded in March 1985 that the small-scale surgery worked as well or better in women with early-stage breast cancer. This was a revolutionary change in a surgical tradition that had persisted for some eighty years. A similar move to less-traumatic surgery occurred in the treatment of soft-tissue sarcomas, malignant tumors that arise in the connective tissues of the body and then spread rapidly. The traditional treatment had often required amputation of the cancerous limb at the nearest joint above the tumor. But in 1986 a fact sheet issued by the National Cancer Institute reported that limb-sparing surgery combined with radiation and drugs was comparable in effectiveness to complete amputation.

The most radical recent development in cancer surgery is the use of surgical techniques to cure metastatic disease as well as the primary cancer site. Over the past decade or more, scientists have discovered that not all tumors metastasize in the same way; some form only a limited number of metastases in the lung, liver, or brain, and these can often be removed by surgeons without further metastasis occurring. Removal of solitary liver metastases in patients with cancer of the colon or rectum has produced long-term cures in about 25 percent of all patients, far exceeding the cure rate of any other treatment. Similarly, removal of lung metastases in patients with soft-tissue sarcomas has cured up to 30 percent of all patients. Surgery is also sometimes used to prevent cancer, as when precancerous polyps are removed to prevent the possibility of cancer in the colon or larynx. President Reagan routinely had tiny polyps removed for laboratory analysis after his 1985 operation for colon cancer, to guard against a recurrence.

Some critics contend that the application of surgery has reached a plateau beyond which it will not progress. Even some surgeons lament that their profession has lost its original intellectual dominance over the treatment of cancer patients.

But surgical refinements will no doubt continue to yield small advances in the war against cancer. It may be absurd to compare the effectiveness of one form of cancer treatment with another, when all of the treatments are essentially complementary. But if doctors were forced to rely on a single weapon against cancer, says Dr. Lucien Israel, a leading clinical researcher in France, most of them would probably choose surgery. It continues to provide the best hope of a cure for the largest number of patients.

RADIOTHERAPY

Radiation, like surgery, is primarily a localized therapy. It uses a beam of radiation rather than a surgeon's knife to destroy a local tumor.

The underlying principle is that radiation is more likely to destroy cancer cells than normal cells. But this is not always the case. Some cancer cells are highly sensitive to radiation, but others are stubbornly resistant.

Unfortunately, radiation can have troublesome side effects. In the short term, it can cause nausea, vomiting, temporary hair loss, fatigue, skin irritations, and loss of appetite. In the long term, it increases the risk of developing another cancer years later. Radiation is not only a cure for cancer, it is also a cause of cancer. It damages normal tissue and can turn it malignant.

The ideal goal of radiation therapy is to destroy a tumor completely while sparing the normal tissue around it. Scientists have searched for decades for a radiation beam of unique physical and biological characteristics that would selectively affect only cancer cells. They have yet to find it. But scientists have made important strides in developing treatments that increase the likelihood of killing tumor cells while inflicting less damage on normal tissue. This remains the principal frontier of modern cancer radiation research.

Radiation therapy got its start in 1896 when X rays, discovered just the year before, were first trained on an inoperable cancer of the stomach. Since then a steady succession of scientific and technical discoveries has led to better understanding of the physical nature of radiation and better ways to deliver it.

Unfortunately, for the first half of the century, radiation equipment was difficult to use, its penetrating powers were relatively slight, and the radiation often caused as much harm as good. Indeed, the scientific literature of the 1920s and 1930s is filled with warnings that radiation therapy is too toxic to use and should be discarded.

But after World War II, radiation therapy began to assume a major role in cancer treatment. A key advance was the introduction, in the 1950s, of more powerful megavoltage equipment, such as the linear electron accelerator and radioactive cobalt sources, which could deliver tumor-killing doses to cancers deep within the body, and could do so without causing the severe skin burns of previous machines.

In the years since, radiation therapists have greatly refined and extended their techniques. They have achieved ever-higher speeds, deeper penetration, sharper delineation of both tumor and radiation beam, and greater sparing of surrounding tissue.

Today, radiation therapists employ a wide variety of radiation sources, including X rays, gamma rays, electrons, and such high-energy subatomic particles as neutrons, heavy ions, and pions, which are still somewhat experimental. The kind of radiation used depends on the type of tumor and its location. Some beams are more effective against superficial tumors since they expend their energy quickly and spare the deeper tissues from damage. Others are more effective against deep tumors and largely spare the surface cells.

The radiation is generally administered from an external machine that shoots a beam into the body. But radioactive implants can sometimes be placed directly in the tumor to deliver their dose at close range, and radioisotopes can sometimes be introduced into the body where they seek out a cancerous target, such as the thyroid gland.

Radiation has thus far proved most effective against the early stages of Hodgkin's disease and against cancers of the cervix, larynx, breast, and prostate, among others. All these are now deemed "radiocurable."

Most often, however, radiation is not used alone but in combination with surgery, on the theory that the strengths of each treatment are complementary. Radiation is most effective against the peripheral cells of tumors but sometimes fails to penetrate to the very center. Surgery, by contrast, has no difficulty removing the core of the tumor but sometimes misses peripheral cancer cells because of the need to preserve vital normal cells adjoining the tumor.

Today, clinical research continues to focus on new ways to enhance radiation's effect on tumors as compared to normal tissues.

One important approach is the use of heavy charged particles to treat cancers that lie too close to vital organs, such as the spinal cord or brain, to be treated by either conventional radiotherapy or surgery without risk of severe damage to the vital organs. The particles' high speed and great energy allow them to penetrate living tissues harmlessly, delivering a high dose of radiation precisely where needed.

At a science writers' seminar in April 1984, Dr. Joseph R.

Castro, of the University of California Medical Center in San Francisco, reported that charged particle irradiation with helium ions had eliminated local spine or skull cancers in 77 percent of a small group of patients who were treated. Even more dramatic results were obtained in treating patients with malignant melanoma of the eye. However, both groups of patients must still be followed for years to determine the long-term effects of the treatment.

American clinicians are also adopting a technique known as intraoperative radiation, first developed in Japan, to deliver radiation directly on the cancer cells. They first remove as much tumor as possible by surgery, then deliver a strong dose of radiation directly on the remaining cancer cells before the surgical incision is closed. This allows a much higher dose of radiation to be delivered without damaging the normal tissue, which is clamped out of the way.

Radiotherapists have steadily refined their precision in locating tumors and directing radiation at them. The latest imaging techniques, such as CAT scans and the newly emerging magnetic resonance imagers, allow the boundaries of a tumor to be defined with a precision never before possible. And computer-controlled direction of the radiation sources allows the beams to be focused with exquisite perfection. As a result, the dose delivered to the tumor is maximized, and the dose spread upon normal tissues is minimized.

Several approaches are being explored to make tumor cells more sensitive to radiation. Over the past five years, for example, hyperthermia, the use of heat to help kill cancer cells, has attracted increasing attention. The heat can be generated by ultrasound, or microwaves, or radio frequencies. By 1984, more than 3,000 patients had been treated with hyperthermia alone, or with a combination of hyperthermia and radiation. Used alone, hyperthermia has proved moderately effective in reducing superficial tumors, on or just under the skin. Used as an adjunct, it has significantly increased the effectiveness of radiation. Scientists at Stanford University reported in 1986 that heat coupled with radiation produced a significant response rate in patients with superficial tumors, such as skin cancers or the chest wall tumors that occur in up to 20,000 breast cancer victims each year. "Today hyperthermia [heat therapy], used in combination with radiotherapy, offers a hopeful option to patients with surface cancers and their physicians when all else has failed," said Dr. Daniel Kapp, director of Stanford's clinical hyperthermia program. Unfortunately, it has proved difficult to attain sufficient heating of deep tumors, or even to measure the heating levels achieved. Hyperthermia seems destined to play a minor but possibly significant role in cancer therapy.

Meanwhile, various drugs are being used to enhance the effect of radiation. Some drugs make tumors more sensitive to radiation; others make the surrounding normal tissue more resistant to damage. Either way, the radiotherapists are moving closer to their goal of killing cancer cells while sparing normal cells.

CHEMOTHERAPY

Chemotherapeutic drugs provided doctors with their first real weapon against cancers that have disseminated widely throughout the body.

The era of modern chemotherapy began in the 1940s with the discovery that nitrogen mustard could cause tumors to shrink and antimetabolites could produce a temporary remission of childhood leukemia. That set off an intensive search for the long-sought "magic bullet against cancer" that would, in one universal sweep through the body, wipe out all cancer cells.

In 1955, the U.S. National Cancer Institute launched a cancer drug development program that soon became one of the nation's biggest cancer efforts. In a prodigious show of brute force testing, the program has acquired and screened more than 700,000 compounds and extracts for antitumor activity. From 1955 to 1975, up to 40,000 agents were screened per year, largely on a random, hit-or-miss basis. For the past decade, a more rational approach has reduced the number screened below 15,000 per year. The end result of this enormous screening effort was a small number of drugs — roughly forty to fifty in all — that have shown significant ability to shrink one or more human cancers for one or more months. This is a "relatively meager armamentarium," in the words of Ezra M. Greenspan, associate chief of medical oncology at the Mount Sinai School of Medicine in New York.

As drug development progressed, the old idea of a single magic bullet gradually faded. A few rare cancers, such as choriocarcinoma, a cancer associated with the placenta in women, and Burkitt's lymphoma, proved vulnerable to single drugs. But other cancers could be conquered only by a combination of drugs. The combinations worked better partly because tumors are a mass of heterogeneous cells, which differ in their sensitivity to various drugs, and partly because drugs often enhance each other's potency. Moreover, by using combinations of drugs, doctors are able to limit their toxic side effects by limiting the amount of any one drug administered.

The most dramatic advance of the 1960s was the development of "sanctuary therapy" to root out the last seeds of cancer from privileged recesses in the body. Conventional drug treatments, for example, could bring about a temporary remission in children with acute lymphocytic leukemia, but, as often as not, tiny seeds of leukemia remained hidden in the central nervous system, safe from the reach of the drugs. The ultimate solution was an additional therapy, combining brain irradiation with drug therapy, that could root the disease out entirely, producing cure rates of 50 to 60 percent in children with acute leukemia. A leading cancer textbook calls this development "one of the great dramas of modern medicine."

The leading milestone of the 1970s was the emergence of adjuvant chemotherapy, which is the use of drugs in conjunction with surgery and radiotherapy. The adjuvant strategy was first applied to childhood cancers in the 1950s and 1960s, but only in the last decade or so has it emerged as a major treatment strategy. The rationale is that drug treatments can pursue and eradicate the last traces of cancer after surgery and radiation have done their best to excise a local tumor. According to a 1984 paper by leading experts at the National Cancer Institute, the demonstration that adjuvant chemotherapy could eradicate microscopic cancer cells "stands as one of the major achievements of the past 10 years."

Estimates of the effectiveness of chemotherapy vary widely. Some leading chemotherapists contend that drugs now cure some

40,000 Americans per year who would otherwise die. But one leading critic insists that the number is closer to 5,000. Either way, it is clear that the vast majority of the 200,000 to 400,000 cancer patients who receive chemotherapy do not get cured by the drugs.

Dr. Emil Frei III, director of the Dana-Farber Cancer Institute of Harvard University, lists thirteen different cancers that have been cured either by chemotherapy alone or by adjuvant chemotherapy in situations where the patient would otherwise die. Most of the cancers are relatively rare, ranging from testicular cancer to certain acute leukemias. Chemotherapy has thus far made little progress against lung or colon cancer, the two major killers in the United States, and only moderate progress against cancer of the breast, the third leading killer.

This lack of effectiveness has caused some doctors to question whether chemotherapy is worth the pain it causes. The drugs are all highly toxic, causing harsh side effects such as nausea, vomiting, diarrhea, temporary hair loss, fatigue, mouth sores, depression, and a loss of resistance to infection.

Unfortunately, the search for new drugs appears to be slowing, partly because of high costs and partly from lack of fresh ideas. George Poste, vice-president for research and development at Smith Kline and French Laboratories, a leading drugmaker, told science writers in April 1984 that "the number of new drugs under development in all therapeutic areas is continuing to fall and cancer therapeutics is no exception." Bruce A. Chabner, director of the division of cancer treatment at the National Cancer Institute, warned in 1982 that the numbers of potential anticancer compounds being identified by the drug screening program "are not encouraging." In early 1987, the National Cancer Institute was preparing to introduce a new testing system to find useful drugs more quickly and accurately. Instead of testing the drugs initially against leukemia in mice, the traditional approach, the new system would first screen the drugs against more than 100 different kinds of human tumor cells growing in test tubes. The new method, due to get started in early 1988, should be far more sensitive than the old one, identifying drugs that are effective against particular tumors even if they would have been dismissed as ineffective against the old mouse leukemia screen. At the same time, the National Cancer Institute was hiring botanists and marine biologists to gather thousands of plants and organisms as a possible source of new anticancer drugs.

The most likely source of advance in the near future is further refinement in the administration of drugs. Indeed, the history of cancer chemotherapy is largely a triumph of applied clinical research. Doctors have taken the drugs with known antitumor activity and greatly enhanced their effectiveness by devising new combinations, new dose levels, and new timing strategies for administering them.

Now they are exploring new ways to administer extra-high doses of drugs for shorter periods of time and new tests to predict which drugs will work best in a particular patient. They are also developing analogues of established drugs that retain their cancer-fighting qualities but have fewer toxic side effects. And they are gaining new insights into how tumors become resistant to drugs, thus allowing drug strategies that can overcome, or even prevent, the development of resistance.

Another emerging technique is the delivery of drugs to limited regions so that they cause maximum damage to the cancer but minimal damage to the rest of the body. One technique is to plant the drugs in the peritoneal cavity or the liver, where they can bathe nearby tumors with up to a thousand times the dose that could safely be delivered through the bloodstream. The drugs can also be infused directly into a region or encapsulated in liposomes whose surface charges determine where they go in the body.

The chief long-term hope is that advances in understanding the fundamental mechanisms by which cancer develops will eventually allow drugs to be tailor-made to disrupt the process. If scientists eventually pinpoint the key molecular differences between cancer cells and normal cells, then drugs may be developed that would home in exclusively on the tumors. At this level, cancer chemotherapy begins to shade into the newer disciplines of genetic engineering and the development of biological compounds that interact with cancer at a molecular level. Indeed, Dr. Chabner and four other experts at the National Cancer Institute recently speculated on what directions cancer chemotherapy might take in the next decade. "It is very likely," they wrote, "that biologic compounds . . . may eventually displace conventional cancer chemotherapy."

BIOLOGICALS

The newest approach in cancer treatment is the search for biological substances, formed naturally in the body or synthesized in the laboratory, that can trigger or augment the body's own defenses against cancer.

The new field represents the reawakening and expansion of a narrower treatment approach known as immunotherapy. Ever since the beginning of the century, scientists have been seeking an immunological cure for cancer, a treatment in which the body's immune system would recognize the difference between tumor cells and normal cells and would mount an attack only against the tumors.

Unfortunately, clinical tests of a variety of substances that were designed to stimulate the immune system showed minimal effect against cancer. A bacterial substance known as BCG, for example, though widely touted as a promising treatment in the late 1970s, has now undergone extensive clinical testing with little evidence of benefit.

In summarizing the results of numerous clinical trials of immunological agents during the 1960s and 1970s, one major cancer textbook concluded: "Most of these failed to demonstrate unequivocal tumor responses attributable to the immunotherapy, leaving the early 1980s to be marked by a certain amount of disappointment and disillusionment in this field."

The chief cause for renewed optimism is that scientists, using an array of new tools associated with the revolution in genetic engineering and recombinant DNA technology, are now able to produce large quantities of biological materials and to design biological weapons that may act selectively against tumor cells instead of simply boosting the body's general immunity levels, as many of the earlier immunological agents did.

Over the past seven years, the National Cancer Institute has identified several groups of biological materials that may eventually be clinically important, the institute reported in September

1984. Some have a direct effect in shrinking tumors; others help the body's normal cells to control cancer cells. In April 1981, the National Cancer Institute established a biological response modifiers program to coordinate laboratory and clinical studies of the new substances.

The first of the new substances to gain wide attention — interferon, a substance produced naturally by the body in response to viral infections — has failed to live up to its initial promise. The substance was widely hailed as a potential cure-all drug when the American Cancer Society invested some $2 million to study its value in patients. But clinical trials have shown limited effectiveness. Only a small percentage of patients have shown a partial decrease in tumor size, and many patients have suffered adverse side effects, including fever, chills, and even hair loss.

A fact sheet issued in September 1984 by the National Cancer Institute reported that a 50 percent decrease in tumor size was seen occasionally in patients with breast cancer, melanoma, and a few miscellaneous solid tumors who were treated with interferon. The response rates were higher in patients with kidney-cell cancer and certain leukemias.

"Interferon is clearly beneficial in some respects," the fact sheet said. "It may not be directly toxic to cancer cells, as conventional drugs are; but it may slow their rate of growth and division so they become sluggish and die."

The institute also noted that interferon was more effective in animals when linked with an anticancer drug, and it suggested that mixtures of different kinds of interferon may prove more effective than a single kind.

"Interferon may indeed prove to have a place in cancer therapy, perhaps as an adjuvant to other modes of therapy rather than as a single treatment," the institute said. "It may prove most helpful in treating cancer that remains after surgery, radiotherapy and/or chemotherapy." Clinical trials have been launched to test interferon in combination with other anticancer agents. In June 1986, the Food and Drug Administration licensed two preparations of interferon for treating hairy-cell leukemia.

Meanwhile, scientists have stepped up their investigations of other proteins that might prove effective against cancer. But many of these, too, promptly ran into the familiar problem of initial exaggerated excitement followed by sober realization of shortcomings. A treatment involving the use of interleukin-2 generated intense publicity and enthusiasm when the National Cancer Institute announced in December 1985 that it had shrunk the tumors of eleven of twenty-five patients with advanced cancer who had failed to respond to other treatments. But in December 1986, the treatment was denounced in an editorial in the *Journal of the American Medical Association* because of its "severe toxicity and astronomical costs" without "commensurate therapeutic benefit." Similarly, a substance known as tumor necrosis factor was considered a promising anticancer treatment when it was put into clinical trials in 1985 but was blamed by some researchers in 1986 for causing weight loss, muscle wasting, shock, and sudden drop in blood pressure.

Another promising biological approach involved the so-called monoclonal, or highly pure, antibodies, which can be designed to seek out, identify, and attack cancer cells on a highly selective basis. Such antibodies can now be produced in larger amounts and with greater specificity than ever before by fusing a cancer cell with a normal antibody-producing cell. The resulting hybrid cell becomes a virtually inexhaustible factory that manufactures large amounts of identical antibody.

Arthur S. Levine, chief of the pediatric oncology branch at the National Cancer Institute, wrote in 1982 that the discovery of how to produce large amounts of monoclonal antibodies ranks as "one of the two recent technical advances in biology — the second being recombinant DNA methodology — which will most influence cancer research in the foreseeable future."

Monoclonal antibodies have already been produced that can specifically detect some of the enzymes, hormones, or antigens produced by certain cancers. In 1986, clinical trials were under way at the Clinical Center of the National Institutes of Health to determine if radiolabeled monoclonal antibodies could detect tumor cells that had spread into the body from colon cancer. The ultimate hope is that monoclonal antibodies might eventually be able to home in on and locate microscopic cancer cells that elude other detection tests, thus providing the most specific test for cancers of various kinds yet devised. The antibodies could be tagged with radioactive materials and followed as they move through the body on an electronic scanner. And beyond mere detection of the cancers lies the possibility of a highly specific treatment. Monoclonal antibodies might be tagged with drugs or radioactive particles that could destroy the tumor at close range, leaving normal cells intact. Indeed, monoclonal antibodies hooked to such biological poisons as diphtheria and ricin toxin have already halted the growth of colorectal cancer cells in animals. Or the monoclonal antibodies can be used alone to trigger destruction of the tumor by the patient's own immune system.

Clinical trials are under way in humans to test the ability of monoclonal antibodies to attack leukemia, lymphoma, and malignant melanoma cells. In preliminary tests, the antitumor effects of these antibodies have not been dramatic, according to the cancer institute, but the antibodies have clearly been able to locate and label the tumor cells.

The early results with biologicals have caused some investigators to exult that an "emerging fourth modality of cancer treatment" may soon claim its place alongside the three conventional therapies. "Never before have so many approaches appeared to be so feasible, practical, and clinically useful," said Robert K. Oldham, a leader of the government's biological response modifiers program, in late 1983.

"Many oncologists would agree that we have reached a plateau in cancer treatment utilizing the three classic modalities of surgery, radiotherapy, and chemotherapy," he said. "The advent of biologicals and biological response modifiers as the fourth modality of cancer treatment will serve to move us from this plateau onto a more effective and more specific therapeutic approach to the treatment of cancer."

Chapter Three

The Chemistry and
the New Understanding of the Brain

By Sandra Blakeslee

Sandra Blakeslee is the West Coast science correspondent of
The New York Times.

The modern revolution in understanding and treating mental illnesses began thirty years ago with what can only be called dumb, blind luck. Luck seemed to rule when researchers then stumbled upon new classes of antipsychotic drugs that drastically changed the course of mental disease. Virtually overnight, the nation's mental hospitals shut their most notorious wards — the "snake pits" — and turned thousands of patients back into the community. While it cannot be said the insane were cured, many patients could begin to cope with life if they took the drugs regularly. The discovery of chemical compounds that could reverse or halt severe mental disorder or alleviate anxiety and depression threw open the door to a new way of thinking about mental illness that is still shaking the foundations of modern psychiatry.

In the 1950s, the mental health field was largely the province

of psychiatrists trained in classical theories of how the unconscious mind can create conflicts that lead to disease. Everything
from schizophrenia to mild depression was seen in this light. In
the 1980s, a different group is leading the study of mental illness.
Trained in the latest concepts of genetics, immunology, pharmacology, and other biological sciences, they are neuroscientists
— "biopsychiatrists" — who feel it is possible to explain human
behavior in terms of the ways molecules fly about in our heads.

Neuroscientists tend to believe the causes of most mental
disorders are rooted not in misguided egos but in biology — in
brain chemicals that don't function properly or in faulty nerve-cell
connections. The antipsychotic, antianxiety, and antidepression
drugs, they argue, work to correct biological imbalances of the
brain. When a healthy person takes an antidepressant drug, he
does not become more cheerful. In their view, autism is not caused
by cold parents. Freudian analysis for schizophrenics is a complete waste of time. Chronic depressions are brain diseases, as
treatable and explainable as diabetes. Separation anxiety syndrome and panic attacks are biological problems, not signs of
weak character or the unconscious desire to manipulate others.
Neuroscientists visualize the brain as a profoundly intricate
feedback system with billions of molecular components and see
mental illness in terms of poorly functioning brain regulatory
mechanisms. As the chemical and physical pathways of the
healthy brain are mapped and described, they say, the biological
causes of mental disorders will surely be found.

Thus the next breakthroughs in mental illness will involve
finding the biological mechanisms that cause the highly orches-
trated brain to lose its balance. Questions involve which brain
cells are altered by which diseases, what events lead to structural
changes that cause mental illness, and how events from the
external world — injuries, infections, stress, even the amount of
daylight — interact with the brain's internal world of inherited
genes that make proteins, hormones, and nerve-cell connections.

The next generation of drugs will not be discovered by
accident. Rather, the modern tools of molecular biology, receptorology, brain imaging techniques, developmental biology, and
genetics that are being turned to the study of the healthy brain

should lead to explanations of the unhealthy brain as well. The next generation of psychotherapies will be short-term treatments that use drugs when appropriate and that dwell more on present attitudes of wellness than past reasons for sickness. In this effort, the interplay between nature and nurture will be better understood and much of the confusion over which mental problems are biological diseases and which are transient psychological problems should be cleared up.

Certainly, experts say, there are situations when a person with a biologically normal brain becomes upset and shows many of the symptoms found in a person who has a mental disorder stemming from imbalances in brain chemistry. Certain kinds of mood swings, sadnesses, anxieties, and phobias can be viewed as "normal," in that they do not reflect an underlying disease state. The environment acts on everyone, and some of life's traumatic events do cause mental distress. The Freudian notion that depression can be caused by a person's turning of anger inward is valid. Ideas, once in the brain, are manipulated by cells and chemicals, thus allowing attitudes to affect mental and physical health. These kinds of mental disturbances in otherwise healthy people are the sorts of problems that respond best to psychotherapy. Drugs are of little value. Upset beliefs, conflicting values, and learned fears can be treated with psychoanalysis, behavior modification, or one of an estimated 250 psychologically based treatments now available to the public.

But many neuroscientists working on mental disorders feel that an extremely high percentage of people who seek treatment for mental distress are suffering from less transient, biological diseases that require drug treatment before psychotherapy can do any good.

There are two general ways people acquire biologically based mental diseases. One way is to be affected by an external agent, something from the outside world that initiates the disease. Chronic stress can upset the brain's balancing act so thoroughly that normal recovery mechanisms are overwhelmed. A disease state sets in. Injury or infection can alter brain function. So-called slow viruses may invade the body and undermine the brain late in life. Drugs, diet, and season of birth influence brain function. A second way involves internal factors, basically, structures and traits that are inherited. Some mental disorders seem to stem from an incomplete "wiring job" of the fetal brain. Any number of things can cause the structural problems (including faulty genes, too much of a hormone, or drugs taken by the mother), but the result is the same. Nerve cells, in very subtle ways, are not connected up in the normal pattern. Other biological structures called receptors and substances called neurotransmitters and peptides may be inherited along abnormal patterns. When these malfunction, mental disorders seem to result.

A central premise of biopsychiatry is that most mental disorders with a biological explanation are manifest in people with a genetic predisposition toward them. Nature and nurture must interact to bring the disease into play. The major mental disorders, such as schizophrenias and manic depressions, have been viewed in this light for many years. But evidence is growing that subtle variations of this interplay — one's genetic constitution as it encounters the environment — could give rise to chronic anxiety, agoraphobia, or panic attacks, school separation anxiety, many kinds of depression, learning disorders, and even sociopathic behavior. Before all this can be proved, however, neuroscientists must learn how the normal brain is wired and how it functions. The task has been called the major medical challenge of the late twentieth century.

The human brain has some 15 billion nerve cells, which potentially make as many connections as there are atoms in the universe. Understanding even the rough outlines of this complex system is no less challenging than demystifying the cosmos. The brain is difficult to see into. Protected by the hardest bone in the body, it operates like a finely tuned orchestra with millions of instruments. Many potent substances are released and then partially reabsorbed in fractions of a second. The amounts involved are vanishingly small. Finding them, one researcher said, is like looking for a greasy needle in a haystack.

Testing substances in the brain is difficult because of a built-in barrier of blood tissues that keeps most substances out. Its complexity is only beginning to be understood. Over a third of our genes are devoted to making substances used by the brain.

Hundreds of thousands of specific brain proteins are continuously manufactured in our heads. Yet we know only a tiny fraction of them. It is certain that some of the undiscovered molecules are involved with mental disorders. Biopsychiatrists face further complications. "There is no clear pathology in pain or depression," said Edward Kravitz, chairman of neurobiology at Harvard University. "It is why all these disorders are so difficult to work with. Pathology of autopsy tissue gives us clues to multiple sclerosis, epilepsy, or Alzheimer's disease, but not to depression or anxiety."

In mental disorders, symptoms are deceptively alike. Loss of appetite, sleeplessness, and nervousness are common signs. But just as a rash can be caused by thirty-eight diseases, there might be thirty-eight biologically different causes of depression. Schizophrenia is certainly a group of diseases. One of the major tasks facing researchers, therefore, is to break the mental disorders into subcategories that are biologically related. Another problem lies in the fact there are no good animal models for most mental disorders. Diseases of the human cerebral cortex — the seat of our abilities to plan and think — are difficult to replicate in lower animals.

Current drugs used to treat mental disorders have unwanted side effects. Their action has been compared to using sledgehammers where lasers are needed. And while there are clues as to how these drugs work, their interaction with brain chemicals and structures is far from understood. To solve these mysteries, researchers in the next few years will follow two interdependent strategies. One involves the fundamental spadework of describing how the brain works, using advanced, noninvasive imaging techniques. The second involves thinking up models of brain structure and function to explain behavior.

In the process of applying neurobiological findings to specific mental disorders, it is certain that new diagnostic techniques, drugs, treatments, and therapies will result.

After decades of surgically peeking and poking into different, small segments of the human brain, today's researchers are about to get a full, three-dimensional, real-time, in-color look at what goes on inside the heads of normal people and of those with mental disorders. The results promise to be spectacular. At last, scientists will be able to relate brain structure with brain function in ways that should go far to explain mental illness. They will do this with the help of powerful imaging techniques that have already been developed. Some are being used to devise anatomical road maps of the brain, while others are working out the traffic patterns of conscious and unconscious thoughts and emotions. When these images are laid side by side and compared in the next few years, whole new descriptions of the brain should emerge.

One set of images comes from devices called CAT scanners, for computer-assisted tomography. These machines, now familiar diagnostic tools in many of the nation's hospitals, are particularly useful in identifying gross abnormalities in brain structure. Tumors, for example, often show up clearly on computer-constructed "slices" of brain tissue. Some mental disorders create recognizable patterns in the brains of those afflicted. CAT scans of one in three schizophrenics, for example, show an abnormality in the spaces between brain lobes. Fluid around the spaces is more prominent. The outer edges of the brain look different, as if shrunken by the disease. Other mental disorders are likely to accompany more subtle anatomical changes that would never show up on a CAT scan. Thus a renewed effort is under way to study the brains of deceased mental patients. The whole brain is cut into 3,000 slices, which are then carefully examined under a microscope for anatomical differences. It is a painstaking process that has shown, for example, that the brains of people with certain learning disorders are "wired" differently from normal brains. The brains of Alzheimer's victims show highly specific cellular damage in an area of the brain called the hippocampus. The damage, researchers say, looks like the destructive path of a tornado cut through a city landscape.

A major goal of mental research in the next few years is to look for specific patterns of cellular abnormalities in the brains of people who had a disease during their lifetimes.

Another technique, called magnetic resonance imaging (MRI), yields detailed pictures of the ridges, folds, and crevices of the brain. Surface landmarks inside the skull can be identified with near-photographic quality. MRI works by picking up signals from the nuclei of elements found in the body. Every organ emits a unique signature of signals. If some mental disorders are associated with too high or too low levels of key elements, such as zinc or magnesium, abnormal patterns should show up on the MRI screen. One theory of Alzheimer's disease, for example, postulates a brain accumulation of aluminum. Such ideas can now be tested. In coming years, MRI will be used to make early diagnoses of diseases like schizophrenia and then follow the course of the illness by observing changes in brain structure. The process of the disease will literally be visualized. New computer techniques are making it possible to take multiple MRI images. It may be possible to image a child's brain in this way every six months or so, actually to observe human brain development. These techniques give fascinating insights into brain anatomy and structure but say nothing about brain chemical and electrical activity — the brain's moving parts.

Positron emission tomography (PET) is a technique that traces brain chemistry. Experiments are under way today, for example, with radioactively tagged glucose — sugar that the brain uses for food energy. As the brain carries out its many tasks, the parts of it that are the most active use up the most sugar. In a PET experiment, the radioactive sugar is injected into the bloodstream of a person who then carries out a mental task — listening to music, writing a letter, or perhaps coping with a painful stimulus. After thirty minutes, the brain is scanned to see where most of the special sugar ended up. The areas with the most radioactivity correlate with where the task was carried out in the brain.

PET glucose scans of schizophrenic patients show they have decreased blood flow to the frontal lobe area of the brain. The sites where antianxiety drugs take effect show up in PET scans of people with general anxiety. People with panic disorders show very different PET scan patterns than do normal people. Young adults who carry the gene for Huntington's chorea can be identified through PET scans long before the disease is overtly manifest. In coming years, PET researchers say they plan to tag radioactively and follow through the brain a wide variety of brain chemicals to see where they concentrate. One such molecule, dopamine, is thought to be overly active in the brains of schizophrenics. PET scans of dopamine activity in the brain promise to shed new light on this class of disorders.

"Keep in mind this won't be easy," said David Pickar, an expert on schizophrenia at the National Institute of Mental Health. "My personal guess is that the schizophrenia syndrome is not a simple overactive dopamine system. It is unbelievably complex and in that complexity we see a poorly controlled dopamine system that goes up and down and is poorly responsive to the environment."

The brain's high-speed traffic patterns are being traced with a new technique called brain electrical activity mapping, or BEAM. It is really an old-fashioned technique — the electroencephalogram — taken to new heights with the help of computers. Up to thirty-two electrodes are placed on the scalp. As a person carries out a mental task, the electrical activity from each electrode is analyzed for its frequency. A number is derived for each electrode, which is then fed into a computerized "map," much as the temperatures from different cities are fed into a national weather map. The great advantage of a BEAM image is that it shows "mental events" moving on the computer screen. As a person listens to music, for example, electrical activity in some areas of the brain is more extensive than in other parts. One can see which parts of the brain respond to a given task in color images that move. Again, people with certain mental disorders show distinctly different brain electrical patterns than do normals. Such testing is just getting under way.

Maps that show "where" the brain thinks may be possible with the help of new cortical imaging techniques. Neuronal activity can be monitored with the help of voltage-sensitive dyes measured with optical recording equipment. Like all maps, the brain's maps are symbolic; people must learn how to read and interpret them, just as they interpret geological maps. The challenge of the future is to understand and interpret the images, which is really a question of how the brain interprets images of the brain.

All these visualizing devices offer complementary images. In the next few years, neuroscientists plan, for the first time, to lay the pictures side by side to get a fuller understanding of mental illness. And as cellular structures and chemical functions are mapped and compared throughout the brain, it will be possible one day to make diagnoses based on imaging techniques. A visit to the PET scanner could tell a patient that he has one kind of schizophrenia and not another or that his panic attacks stem from an imbalance in one brain chemical.

Early symptoms of some diseases might be found with imaging techniques — before psychotic behavior sets in — thus allowing early treatment or perhaps prevention with drug therapies.

MENTAL DISORDERS

In the past few years, neurobiologists have developed a fabulous arsenal of tools and models for looking at how the human brain works. Some seek to explain how nerve connections are laid down, while others describe the great variety of chemical messengers that constantly flit through the brain along specific pathways. Many of the breakthroughs in the understanding of mental disorders will stem directly from these models as they are applied to specific diseases of mood, personality, and emotion.

The most general model holds that all information processing in the brain involves neurons "talking" to one another at synapses. Molecules called neurotransmitters move across the synapse — a tiny gap between nerve cells — to land on specific chemical sites, called receptors, on a neighboring nerve cell. Sometimes some of the neurotransmitter is reabsorbed by the releasing cell, just as a sponge mops up excess liquid. Or enzymes in the synapse break down neurotransmitters. Once the right amount of transmitter is delivered to the neighboring cell, however, "information" has been passed. Receptors on the receiving cell cause channels in its membrane to open. Each cell has hundreds of thousands of these channels, or protein portholes, that regulate its electrical activity. Charged particles, called ions, of hydrogen, potassium, sodium, or calcium move through the membrane, setting up a small electric impulse in the stimulated neuron. The stimulus turns the brakes on or off — it inhibits or excites — by causing that cell to release its own transmitters. The process continues, cascade fashion, throughout a pathway until some goal is met.

In a healthy person, these chemical messages are governed by internal "rheostats," or feedback mechanisms that maintain a balance. A correct number of receptors and transmitters are maintained. Neurons do not overproduce or underproduce messages. Pulses are brief and precise. With this model in mind, scientists have been able to identify some sixty neurotransmitters and nearly 100 receptor molecules in the brain. Many are implicated with mental disorders. Epilepsy, for example, is associated with the overproduction of a neurotransmitter called "GABA." Obsessive-compulsive behavior is associated with a deficiency of the neurotransmitter serotonin. Hyperactivity is related to an underactive dopamine system. The spinal fluid of people who commit suicide contains an unusually low concentration of a substance (5-HIAA) that is a major breakdown product of serotonin. It may be that serotonin-releasing neurons are for some reason less active in people inclined to suicide.

Up to now, the identification of neurotransmitters and their receptors has been hit or miss. Most were discovered by accident. Some were purified from the brain tissue of thousands upon thousands of animals killed in slaughterhouses. Others are substances long known to exist but only now being recognized as transmitters, including some common amino acids that are building blocks of proteins. What is different about the research of the next few years is that methods are now available to identify such molecules methodically and purposefully. And this establishes a whole new ball game in the search for biological mechanisms of mental disorders. The new methods involve tools of molecular biology that cleverly make cells relinquish their secrets. Specifically, to know a cell is to know its proteins. Proteins drive a cell's metabolism, supply it with energy, and build its internal structures and membranes. They interact in a nerve cell in ways that allow the cell to communicate with other cells. Neurotransmitters, receptors, and other important brain-messenger molecules are all proteins.

But here's the rub. Most of the really interesting proteins in brain cells — and likely many that are involved in mental illness

— are produced in such minuscule amounts that researchers have no hope of isolating and purifying them by conventional methods (such as grinding up thousands of sheep brains and extracting a speck of the interesting protein). An alternative way to get at these proteins has been found. Each protein is the product of a gene found in the brain-cell nucleus. If the gene that makes a protein is known, it is a straightforward job to work out the exact properties of the protein.

Using recombinant DNA methods, genes can be isolated, and researchers have begun the enormous task of identifying the ones that are active in brain-cell tissue. Already, a small handful of previously unknown brain proteins have been identified.

The next step will be to test the functions of the mystery proteins in laboratory animals to see if they affect behavior. Based on these methods, researchers say they expect to find up to 700 neurotransmitters and many times more receptors. As such molecules are hunted down and tested, new explanations of mental disorders will inevitably come about. For example, sleep disturbances are a basic characteristic of many mental illnesses. The neurochemistry of sleep may turn up important clues about depression and mania and how visual centers are affected by these disorders.

"This work is really just beginning," said Katherine Bick, deputy director of the National Institute of Neurological and Communicative Disorders and Stroke in Bethesda, Maryland. "But all these proteins must be doing something. You can imagine that even very small changes produce massive behavioral kinds of anomalies."

Another approach to understanding mental disorder involves developmental biology. Scientists now know that the human embryonic brain produces excess neuronal connections. Before and around the time of birth, a natural pruning occurs. Vast numbers of neurons compete for position and millions die off. Some theorists say this process can run amok, and that may explain certain mental disorders. If, for example, too many or too few neurons occupy a given area, later mental functioning could be impaired. Another hypothesis holds that hormonal influences around puberty cause the brain to again "rewire," and that some types of schizophrenia could result from errors in this process. Careful sectioning of human brain tissue is expected to shed light on these ideas and perhaps explain some mental disorders.

Geneticists are also getting involved in mental health research, and their contributions in coming years will be major. Family studies have shown there are clear genetic factors in many mental disorders, including depression, anxiety, alcohol abuse, and schizophrenia. Identical twins, for example, may develop the same type of schizophrenia even if raised apart. But the precise risk of inheriting such disorders is unclear. Unanswered questions before geneticists include: Is shyness in early childhood related to adult phobia? Is suicide familial? Is there a relationship between drug abuse, other addictive behaviors, and psychiatric disorders?

"We will have valid markers of genetic vulnerability to particular psychiatric illnesses," said Eliot Gershan of the National Institute of Mental Health. "These will serve two purposes. They will subdivide illnesses into distinct biological syndromes, and they will give us very strong clues as to what underlies the development of the syndrome."

Recently, researchers localized the abnormal gene responsible for Huntington's chorea, which causes profound mental and physical deterioration in its victims, and for Alzheimer's disease, which causes severe dementia. From this, they plan to develop tests to screen family members who might inherit these diseases. Such gene markers serve as proxies for hidden genes. They are simply bits of DNA that lie near a gene implicated in a disease. Researchers are confident that genetic markers will be found for every mental disorder. While many genes are likely to be involved in mental diseases such as manic depression — wild mood swings from euphoria to despair — it should be possible to test individuals with a family history of the disease to determine if they have inherited genes associated with the problem. Or the second child in a family that already has one child with a given disease can be tested to see if he or she also carries the defective gene or is predisposed to develop the disease. Illnesses will be divided into distinct, multigenic biological syndromes.

Psychiatrists today have a difficult job in diagnosing mental disorders, said Erminio Costa, chief of the laboratory of preclinical pharmacology at St. Elizabeth's Hospital in Washington, D.C. "The big thing that has to happen is to find a way to characterize mental diseases in an objective way." Diagnostic tests using genetic markers, Dr. Costa said, will be the way to go.

Neurobiology has spawned a whole new field called receptorology that also promises to revolutionize mental health research. All psychoactive drugs act directly or indirectly on receptors — those proteins with specific recognition sites for neurotransmitters. Some drugs plug up receptor sites, while others block the "mopping up" ability of contiguous nerve cells. Receptors are clearly changed in a variety of psychiatric illnesses, but it is not yet known if the changes are a cause or an effect of the disease. For example, people with manic depression show a decreased density of acetylcholine receptors. Huntington's patients have obvious changes in several receptor systems. Receptor mapping techniques are brand-new, said Michael Kuhar of the National Institute on Drug Abuse. "So much has happened in the last five years. It's like a moonshot."

With new receptor mapping techniques in hand, Dr. Kuhar and other "receptorologists" have begun finding multiple receptors for some neurotransmitters. Thus, there are now dopamine-1 and dopamine-2 receptors that seem to have different functions. Receptor experts say there may turn out to be three or four closely related receptors for each neurotransmitter. The picture is getting more complicated, to be sure, but it is also more accurate. Entire brain receptor maps are being redrawn. One group, for example, is mapping all the body's anxiety receptors. An endogenous valium-like substance in our bodies or an anxiety-provoking substance has been implicated with these receptors.

The next step will be to image newly found receptor molecules in the brains of living mental patients. This can be done before and after drug treatment to see how receptors respond. This work closely parallels another new subfield in neurobiology involving molecules called peptides. Peptides are small proteins found throughout the nervous system that exert spectacular effects on the mind and body. Quite literally, a new peptide is being discovered every week. The body's own "morphine," for example, is a peptide. A peptide that attaches to the receptors sensitive to the street drug PCP have been found, suggesting that the brain produces a natural psychogenic substance. Marvels await in peptide chemistry.

Peptides seem to act both like neurotransmitters and hormones (although they work slowly like hormones and not quickly like transmitters). Recently it has been shown that some neurons contain both "classical" transmitters and peptides. In some instances the peptides seem to support the action of the transmitters. Such interaction may have wide-ranging implications for mental diseases. A peptidelike substance, for example, has been found in dopamine-rich neurons implicated in schizophrenia. The peptide neurotensin may modulate dopamine release and thus also play a role in the disease.

Peptides have aroused the attention of biopsychiatrists because peptides tend to be found in the parts of the brain that deal with emotions and feelings. When peptides are administered to animals, profound behavioral changes are common. The animals may become paralyzed, paranoid, or petrified. Thus a major thrust of research in the next few years will involve relating peptides to psychiatric disorders. Alzheimer's victims have a reduced level of the peptide somatostatin. And depressed patients have been found to have elevated levels of a peptide called CRF in their spinal fluid. The peptide may be "in overdrive," researchers say.

In yet another investigative strategy, researchers plan to study the biological rhythms of brain chemicals. There is compelling evidence that some kinds of depression result when hormones are secreted at the wrong time of day. Greater understanding of these daily or seasonal rhythms is expected to assist in the treatment of several mental disorders.

Finally, the search for viruses implicated in mental disease continues. Viruses are known to damage selectively the central nervous system. Polio virus, for example, attacks anterior horn cells in the spinal cord. Herpes virus can damage the temporal lobe in the brain. Both Alzheimer's disease and some types of schizophrenia may be caused by viruses, according to some researchers, and could be eradicated one day with vaccines.

THERAPIES AND DRUGS

As findings flow from these various research strategies, new therapies and treatments are certain to follow. All the drugs used today for treating schizophrenia, depression, and anxiety achieve their therapeutic ends by affecting only a handful of the best-known transmitters and receptors. Most of these drugs have unpleasant to serious side effects.

Next, "it will be possible to sculpt a drug selectively to one of its receptors," said Solomon Snyder, a neuroscientist at Johns Hopkins University. "All the peptides are interesting and it is likely we have all the methodologies we need for getting new drugs based on them. Once you know the chemistry of a substance, you look for drugs to block its formation or destruction at a receptor." If a transmitter is out of kilter, for instance, a new drug may work by modulating a co-transmitter instead of the transmitter itself. Drugs that mimic or prevent the action of peptides would be powerful pharmacological tools.

Such drugs will be far more precise in the ways they affect the feedback circuits of the brain. They will alter the way brain chemicals are timed or amplified instead of blocking their action entirely. And drug interaction with neuronal circuits will be more important than action at the synapses. "We may soon find whole new classes of drugs," Dr. Snyder said. "There may be diseases or system complexes that we don't think about now. Maybe one day we could treat extreme shyness."

New computer imaging techniques are expected to help pharmacologists design new drugs with less guesswork. Imaginary molecules can be manipulated on a screen as if they hung in midair. "It will be possible to develop some rational ideas about drug design," Dr. Bick said. "You can get a better feel with computer graphics. You can see the molecule, turn it around and put it together with what we know about receptors." Mental health experts expect many such developments to come primarily from small genetic engineering companies instead of the traditional pharmaceutical giants.

New forms of psychosurgery are around the corner. But instead of taking tissue out, as in a lobotomy, surgeons are putting substances back into mentally diseased brains. In so-called brain transplants, grafts of missing proteins might be inserted into an affected brain region. A neuronal circuit may need only a gentle "kick" to work normally again. Alzheimer's patients may have acetylcholine "pumps" refilled as regularly as diabetics take insulin shots. Depressed patients might have peptide pumps.

Where does this leave traditional psychotherapy? Is all mental distress going to be handled in future with shots or pills?

According to even the most pro-biological experts in the field of mental health research, the answer is no, of course not. People will always develop mental problems that are not rooted in "wrong molecules" or "bad genes." Many depressions, phobias, and anxious states result from life stresses that are best treated by psychological counseling. Even after a biologically based mental disorder is successfully treated with a drug, there is need for psychotherapy, said Benjamin S. Bunney of Yale University's psychiatry department, a need to unlearn the feeling of helplessness. Neurobiology and psychotherapy can work together. Take Tourette's syndrome, for example, in which young people, starting around age five, develop abnormal motor movements and swear and curse at everything. "For a long time this was treated with psychotherapy," Dr. Bunney said, "but it never helped." Eventually doctors began to treat the disorder with an antipsychotic drug, and patients got much better. But they still weren't cured.

"You can treat with drugs," Dr. Bunney said, "but these people still need psychotherapy. While sick, they were ostracized by peers, picked on by teachers, or punished by parents. That is the role of psychotherapy, to try to undo that. It makes them feel good about themselves and gives them self-confidence." Things like self-confidence, self-image, and ability to relate to others are not going to be biochemically or electrophysiologically understood "for centuries probably," Dr. Bunney said. Even if biopsychiatrists learn the underlying biological process of what causes delusion, the patient is still left with what it meant to him and how society treated him.

Psychotherapy is moving away from classical schools into new directions based on cognitive, behavioral, or interpersonal treatments. A recent survey of clinical psychologists, for example, ranked Sigmund Freud third (behind Carl Rogers and Albert Ellis) among important figures in psychotherapy. People can no longer afford years of open-ended psychotherapy, said Arthur Freeman of the Center for Cognitive Therapy at the University of Pennsylvania. "We have reached a point where people come in and ask the therapist, 'What will you do? How much will it cost? How long will it last? What studies do you have that show me what you do works?' "

Psychologists and psychiatrists, Dr. Freeman said, will be far more accountable in future. Mental health agencies and insurance companies are demanding that therapists prepare quarterly treatment plans and that they share these with the patients. Goals of short-term therapy are set forth from the beginning. Studies of how well various therapies work are under way, to compare the efficacy of different approaches. For example, short-term structured therapy aimed at treating misinterpretations and misconceptions has been extraordinarily effective in phobias, anxiety, and eating disorders, according to Dr. Aaron Beck, also of the University of Pennsylvania. Many panic disorders apparently stem from a catastrophic misinterpretation of body sensations. The sensations are biologically real and run in families, said Dr. Beck, but people lose the ability to reason about their problem. "We can now take someone with a biological or genetic component," he said, "and can revert the problem psychologically, without drugs." Studies comparing drug treatment as opposed to therapy alone will help tease apart nature and nurture.

"The excitement today lies in the attitude that there is really nothing you can't ask," said Dr. Katherine Bick. "To me, this is what sets the stage for a real revolution. You open up the windows and don't see a horizon that will limit you. Then the stage is set for great leaps forward." The argument of whether mental illnesses derive from nature or nurture, she said, "persists as a measure of our ignorance. When we understand nature, we'll be able to fit nurture into it."

Chapter Four

Organ Transplantation:
From the Experiment to the Routine

By David R. Zimmerman

David R. Zimmerman is the author of several medicine and environment articles and books, including Rh: The Intimate History of a Disease and Its Conquest *and* To Save a Bird in Peril.

The baby suddenly was visible in the surgical cut in her mother's abdomen.

Doctors in the delivery room at the University of California Medical Center at San Diego watched the baby's and the mother's heartbeats on electronic monitors that looked like TV sets. But they watched the mother's heart rate with far more than a routine concern.

"Can her heart stand the stress of surgical childbirth?" was everyone's unspoken question.

This was the reason for their concern: the heart beating in the twenty-three-year-old woman's chest was not the heart she had been born with. It was a transplanted heart, from a twenty-three-year-old accident victim, that had been given to her four years before — after a tumor damaged her own heart and threatened her life.

Her doctors were particularly worried because this woman was the first heart transplant recipient to carry a pregnancy to term. What is more, the heart now supporting her circulatory system and life, and her baby's, had not belonged to a woman.

No man's heart had ever before withstood the rigors of pregnancy, labor, and the delivery of a baby.

The heart itself, and the sutures and scar tissue connecting it into the young mother's body held securely. The delivery, by itself, was uneventful. Mother and baby — a 7-pound, 1-ounce daughter who was named Sierra — later were reported to be doing well.

The heart had expanded considerably in size during pregnancy in order to pump more blood — as a woman's heart normally does — even though the normal nerve connections between heart and brain were lacking. Reported the mother's doctor, Thomas Key: "Her transplanted heart experienced the same changes during pregnancy as a female heart would, although she doesn't have the normal neurotransmission from brain to heart."

The transplanted male heart seems to have responded appropriately, on its own, to the stress of supporting an additional living being, the baby in the womb.

Beyond its warm human appeal, this case reflects a key change in organ transplant surgery, the replacement of a diseased organ with a homologous organ from a living or newly dead human donor. Organ transplantation is moving out of the realm of scientific experimentation. It is becoming — and before the turn of the century will be solidly established as — a medical practice. It will have become a technically routine lifesaving method.

Organ transplantation, after a half century of research and development, is thus coming of age. Its lifesaving benefit is spreading outward from the handful of research hospitals where the surgical techniques first were developed. It is — or soon will become — available in hundreds of hospitals around the world.

Given the monumental problems of transplant surgery, which are by no means all resolved, this is incredible progress. The very first successful organ transplant — a kidney taken from one identical twin and sutured into the other — took place in 1954, in Boston.

There now have been over 85,000 kidney transplants, world-wide, according to the American Council on Transplantation (ACT), a national public policy organization set up to monitor the progress and help solve some of the great social problems that have been raised by the method's growing success. Some kidney transplant recipients, ACT says, now have been sustained in life for over thirty years with their donor organs. Well over 90 percent of all kidney transplant operations now are successful, meaning that the organ functions in the recipient for at least a year.

The liver, which is a larger and far more intricate organ, has been a greater challenge to surgeons: Only in 1967 did surgeon Thomas Starzl and his tight-knit team of co-workers perform the first successful human liver transplant.

Over 2,500 of these operations have now been done. The majority were for children who faced certain death because their own livers were failing to function owing to birth defects or disease. One of the transplant recipients, operated on when she was about five years old, already has passed her seventeenth birthday. Two-thirds of liver transplants, ACT says, are successful.

The human heart first was successfully transplanted in 1967, by the South African surgeon Christiaan Barnard. Close to 4,000 hearts have since been transplanted. More than three-quarters of these operations are successful now — and one recipient is still going strong after eighteen years.

More recently, doctors have started to transplant the heart and a lung together, for persons whose lungs are fatally diseased. This is technically more feasible than transplanting only the lung. Over 120 of these operations have now been performed in the United States. About half of these heart-lung transplants are successful, and one patient now has survived with a heart-lung graft for over three years.

The other major vital organ that has occupied transplanters' attention is the pancreas — which has a tiny area of cells, called the islets of Langerhans, that produce insulin. This vital hormone facilitates the body's storage and use of sugar.

Over 500 pancreas transplants have been attempted. Over a third of these grafts now survive a year or longer; one patient has survived for more than five years. Despite recent progress, however, pancreas transplantation still is considered experimental surgery. "We fully expect [it] to stand the test of time," pioneer pancreatic transplant surgeon Dr. Robert J. Corry, of the University of Iowa College of Medicine, said in 1987. "We have every reason to believe it will prove to be successful in [relieving] the diabetic state." Meanwhile, some novel modifications, in which only the islet cells are transplanted, are being developed.

Several major problems have stood in the way of wide use of transplantation. Some of these problems are now largely resolved; others are a continuing challenge to doctors and society as a whole.

A major bar has been immunologic incompatibility between the recipient and the available donor organs. The biologic identity of individual human beings, and of other members of the animal kingdom, is expressed through a set of several proteins, called antigens, on the surface of most body cells, and a corresponding set of antibodies that will attack and destroy antigenic substances, including living cells that are different from the individual's. In this way, each individual's antibodies recognize most other persons' body tissues as "non-self," and attack and destroy them.

Most donor organs — whether they are kidneys, hearts, or livers — thus are recognized by the recipients as not belonging, as something foreign to themselves. The white blood cells activate the recipient's immune system, which tries to destroy the lifesaving transplant! (In some cases, what may be worse, antibodies in the transplanted organ attack the recipient's body. This graft-versus-host disease often is fatal.)

The first strategy that was mounted to overcome these rejection problems was to perform transplants only between identical twins. Because they arise from the same fertilized human egg, identical twins' immune systems recognize each other as self — and transplants between them usually are well accepted.

While not perfect matches, family members who are not twins often are more compatible, immunologically, than people who are not blood relatives. So parents and siblings may be the most suitable donors for the great majority of would-be recipients who lack an identical twin.

In practice this borrowing of organs between family members has been useful only for kidneys. Each of us normally has two of these organs — which control the levels of vital chemicals and water in the body and filter wastes out of the bloodstream so they can be excreted through the bladder as urine. One kidney can provide normal function. So it is relatively safe to have one kidney removed surgically, for transplantation, to sustain a loved one's life.

For livers, hearts, and other one-of-a-kind organs, however, this borrowing from the living cannot be done. The need for these organs — and for kidneys, for the many persons who lack an immunologically compatible and willing family donor — is great, but the only source is organs taken from the bodies of people who have just died. Major scientific, logistic, legal, and ethical changes have been required to make compatible "cadaver donor organs," as they sometimes are called, available to would-be recipients whose lives hang in the balance.

A major advance was made by Paul Teraseki, who is a professor of surgery at the University of California Medical School at Los Angeles. He reported, in the 1960s, that several sets of genes determine immunologic "self" recognition. Tests that he devised showed how close, immunologically speaking, needful patients and dead or dying potential donors may be. By entering data for patients and cadaver donors into a computer data bank, and analyzing this information, surgeons could find the best matches between their patients and the organs available at the moment of need. This testing in the HLA (human leukocyte antigen) system continues to be used to match transplant recipients and organ donors.

The HLA testing, however, does not always locate a suitable match. Sometimes apparently well-matched grafts fail. The other course researchers have pursued to overcome graft rejection is to give special drugs to damp down or repress the immune response. A succession of these immunosuppressive drugs have been used. But even into the present decade, none was impressively effective.

A recent new drug, cyclosporine, which was approved for

clinical use in the United States only in 1983, has markedly improved matters. Cyclosporine is very effective. Through its use, the transplant success rate for some organs has been doubled, or better, at some transplant centers. The advent of cyclosporine, in fact, is regarded by doctors as one of the key elements in transforming transplantation from an experiemental to a clinical procedure.

As more and more cyclosporine has been used, it unfortunately has been found to have some shortcomings of its own. Perhaps most threatening, researchers from Stanford University, among others, have reported that transplant patients who are on maintenance doses of cyclosporine suffer kidney damage as a result.

In reporting these findings to the *New England Journal of Medicine*, nephrologist Bryan D. Myers warns: "Any benefit derived from reduced rejection of . . . transplants may be more than offset over the long term by chronic kidney damage induced by the cyclosporine."

The advent of cyclosporine clearly has not ended the quest for safe and effective immunosuppressive drugs and other agents to prevent transplant rejection. But dramatically improved one-year survival rates since its introduction indicate that a fair piece of the problem has been solved.

A more immediate — and more grim — problem is that of finding and obtaining cadaver donor organs. For someone to live, someone must die, and in a manner that allows doctors to "recover" the transplantable organs.

The best candidates are relatively young, healthy persons who have died suddenly, or been killed. Since next-of-kin permission and complex arrangements typically are required, the best candidates are persons who have died in major hospitals, where their bodies can continue to be maintained by life-support systems, even though their brain waves are flat, signifying death.

In the United States, with a population of more than 240 million, it has been calculated that there are about 25,000 such brain-death cases each year. To obtain the organs, explains organ procurement director Donald W. Denny of the University of Pittsburgh liver transplant program, over 180 organ procurement teams have been established across the nation. When they learn of a dying or brain-dead potential donor, they enter the relevant information in a computer data base that serves to alert transplanters of the availability of organs suitable for their patients.

When a match is made, a scramble ensues. The patient has to be called to the hospital, if he or she is waiting at home for a transplant, and has to be prepared for surgery.

The organs, meanwhile, are taken surgically from the donor's body and prepared for transport to the (often) distant city where they are needed. The organs are chilled, to retard degeneration, and may be perfused with fluids.

The time window for transporting a donor organ and restarting it in the recipient's body, in practice, is still very brief. When simply chilled, ACT says, organs must be reimplanted within these times:

> kidneys, 48–72 hours
> livers, 8–12 hours
> hearts, 3–4 hours
> heart-lungs, 1–2 hours
> pancreases, 8–24 hours.

One donor obviously can provide several organs, and so sustain several lives as a final gift to others. But many legal, ethical, and religious objections must be overcome in order for this to be possible. In the United States and some other countries it already is legal for individuals to carry brief "wills," called uniform donor cards, in their wallets or pocketbooks that grant their organs to others. Where no such direction can be found, the next of kin must grant permission — and if the kin cannot be found or refuses permission, the organs cannot be obtained.

If death is defined as the cessation of heartbeat, or the time that the body grows cold, it may be too late to recover usable organs. So states and other governmental jurisdictions are changing the definition of death. According to the newer standard, once higher mental activity has ceased, so that the electroencephalograph (EEG) waves are flat, the individual cannot recover, and thus is "brain dead," even though the heart beats on, with the help of a life-support system. Acceptance of this new definition of death facilitates the recovery of viable donor organs from individuals who have been sustained in their terminal illnesses by life-support systems. Thirty of the states in the United States now have passed laws that define death as the complete and irreversible cessation of all brain function.

However, even in countries where these options are legal, only a small percentage of brain-dead injury victims in fact provide organs for transplant. The U.S. government says only about 15 percent of the 25,000 persons who reach this state each year do so.

Given the growing need for these organs, medical ethicist Arthur L. Caplan, recently of the Hastings Center at Hastings-on-Hudson, New York, has suggested that the law be changed: he suggests that hospitals not be allowed to turn off life-support systems after a patient suffers brain death until they have contacted a family member or legal guardian to request donor organs.

"In view of the desperate needs of those who are now awaiting organs, and the large number of persons who will be able to benefit from transplantation in the years to come," Caplan says, "the loss of this freedom [to turn off the life-support system without asking for the organs] would seem to be a small price to pay."

Some state legislators agree with Caplan. By 1987, fifteen states had passed laws requiring hospitals to solicit organ donations from next of kin.

The growing availability of transplantation — and the life salvage it offers — thus requires profound changes in people's beliefs and the laws through which they find social expression. In cultures that view the removal of organs as defiling the dead, it is obvious that transplant programs cannot be carried out.

The other side of the coin is that some laws must be rewritten to prevent transplant patients' needs from subverting moral sensibility and the law. One such area is the sale of donor organs — of a kidney by a living donor, for example, or of cadaver organs that an individual might "sell" during life for delivery at death, or that the family or unscrupulous other people might find ways to attain. At worst, a commerce in human organs could be an open invitation to murder.

To prevent such destructive eventualities, medical and legal authorities have taken a strong stand against the sale of human organs. In a report to the U.S. Congress, for example, the assistant secretary for health, Dr. Edwin N. Brandt, Jr., said: "We are opposed to the sale of human organs, because we believe that such activity is immoral, and goes against the principles of medical ethics. We are particularly concerned about those persons willing to sell their organs who may not fully understand the serious consequences of their action."

The sale of human organs and tissues now is forbidden in the United States by federal law.

Human organs nevertheless are, inescapably, scarce and limited resources. How to obtain and how to allocate them continue to be pressing — and unresolved — questions.

These concerns are focused, for the moment, on livers, since the need for this organ is the most acute. (Patients whose natural kidneys have failed can be kept alive indefinitely on artificial kidney machines, or dialyzers. Patients whose hearts are failing still have relatively few transplant options, because only about ninety surgical teams are willing and able to perform heart transplants.) The need for livers is particularly compelling because many of the most suitable patients, medically speaking, are very young children. For them, the availability of a suitable donor organ may mean the difference between immediate death and the possibility of a full and essentially normal and productive life.

Many distraught parents of these children have gone on TV and appealed to the public through the press for a donor. Some have been rewarded when their appeal became known to grieving parents who had just lost a child with a comparable-sized liver in an accident or through disease.

The procurement computer network — called OPTN (for Organ Procurement and Transplantation Network) — that keeps track of needy recipients and incipient donors throughout the United States uses a code system to rate the urgency of need. A "Status 0" means the patient is in imminent risk of death and has a priority for any usable liver that becomes available.

As of 1987, forty-five hospitals in the United States were performing liver transplants. Other hospitals are gearing up to do so. But because of the tremendous expense of training the surgeons and other personnel, and providing space and supplies for this surgery, the cost, for the moment, is likely to exceed the fiscal return — despite the high prices that patients are charged. The fear of constantly losing money has restrained hospitals from starting liver transplant programs.

One major need for the immediate future, then, is the training and equipping of many additional transplant teams. The related great need is to find ways to deal with the enormous cost.

The figures are frightening: In the United States, recently, the average cost of a liver transplant was $267,000; in some cases the bill has been much higher.

Few families can afford these fees. In some communities, civic groups have stepped in to help families raise the money. But more organized forms of community help are needed.

The recent decision by government health officials in the United States that liver transplantation represents acceptable medical practice — not clinical experimentation — in several rare, lethal children's liver diseases has had a major social consequence that is being felt around the world, as other governments and medical bodies arrive at similar decisions: Medical insurance must begin to offer insurance coverage for liver graft surgery.

In the United States, the federal government now pays for liver transplants for infants and children with some rare, deadly diseases. A national debate was in progress, in the late 1980s, as to whether, and if so how, society should support this surgery for people who lack the necessary personal resources or private or group insurance.

Many of the major American private health insurance companies have started to offer this coverage. The large employee health plans are following suit — but more slowly. They say that if they underwrite transplantation surgery too soon, before enough surgeons have been trained to the task, many patients will die in botched operations.

The question is, what will liver transplants cost insurance policyholders? One recent estimate in the United States is that each policy will have to be increased five to ten dollars per year, just to cover the few children's diseases for which this operation is the only hope for survival.

As techniques improve, however, there may be more and more illnesses, including drug-induced and viral hepatitis and liver cancer, for which transplantation may be the sole hope for survival. Many more of the costly transplants then would be needed each year — and insurance premiums could be expected to rise accordingly.

The social dilemma becomes clearest in the case of liver damage (cirrhosis and hepatitis) caused by intemperate use of alcoholic beverages. This is the "most common" form of fatal liver disease in the United States, the National Institutes of Health (NIH) has pointed out. Should these patients be given — and should society pay for — liver transplants?

Recent guidelines issued by NIH indicate that only reformed alcoholics who will abstain from drinking are appropriate candidates for transplants. "Only a small proportion of alcoholic patients with liver disease would be expected to meet [this] rigorous criterion," the NIH guidelines say.

Knowledgeable physicians say, however, that some unreformed, but rich, alcoholics have sought — and obtained — liver transplants. If rich alcoholics can pay for this care, then is society obliged to provide transplants for less well-off unrepentant drunks?

Many people, citing precepts of social justice, say yes. A controversial negative answer has come from a physician and medical ethicist, Hugo T. Engelhardt, Jr., of the Baylor College of Medicine. He sees the allocation of scarce transplant resources as one of the ever-commoner "scientific debates with heavy political and ethical overlays" that cannot be resolved on wholly scientific or on wholly moral grounds.

"In the background of these determinations," Dr. Engelhardt says, "is a set of moral judgments regarding equity, decency, and fairness, cost-benefit trade-offs, individual rights, and the limits of state authority."

In his view, society cannot force members of a democracy to pay for transplantation or other costly medical procedures if they do not wish to. He justifies this by drawing a "painful line" between what he calls unfortunate and unfair outcomes in life.

He says that the need for a heart transplant is an unfortunate natural circumstance. But if society does not wish to pay for it, it is not unfair, even though some people will die for want of the operation.

"To live with circumstances [that] we must acknowledge as unfortunate, but not unfair, is the destiny of finite men and women — who have neither the financial nor the moral resources of gods and goddesses," Dr. Engelhardt says.

These issues have been carefully considered by a federal advisory panel on organ transplants, appointed by President Ronald Reagan. The panel proposed, in 1986, that no more than 10 percent of kidney transplants performed in the country be provided to persons who are not U.S. residents. Nonresidents also should be given lowest priority for heart and liver transplants, the panel said.

The panel proposed, as its recommendation, that the federal government oversee a national transplant network, which would find organ donors and also guarantee that "inability to pay" would not prevent any American from receiving a needed heart or liver. The panel envisioned a transplant network that would include all private, nonprofit agencies that find and distribute organs to hospitals across the country. The network then would be able to enforce guarantees of fairness in donor organs' use.

The panel's proposals were received coolly by the Reagan administration, which said it would prefer that the private sector, rather than the federal government, operate and supervise organ distribution and transplant surgery.

Clearly, the societal debates over transplantation are only beginning. On the other hand, successful technologic advances such as transplantation rarely are abandoned. They are integrated into social (and, of course, medical) practice, in a pragmatic and functional way.

One form of accommodation is technologic refinement. It may, for example, be possible to get the same result with less cost: It may not be necessary to transplant an entire pancreas, in order to obtain the life-sustaining benefit this organ provides. Researchers have been searching for ways to separate the crucial insulin-producing islet cells from the rest of the pancreas — which they now know how to do — and then transplant them, without major surgery, into a recipient.

Recent experiments in dogs foreshadow success in this endeavor. Surgeons at Mount Carmel Mercy Hospital in Detroit, Michigan, have reported, for example, that they can cure diabetes in dogs by injecting donor-dog islet cells into pockets created surgically between the outer and inner layers of one kidney. The islet cells appear to survive and function better at this unusual, and unnatural, location than they do when transplanted into other sites in the body.

The Detroit researchers did not use immunosuppressive drugs. They do not know why the islet cells survived and functioned, producing insulin, in the dogs' kidneys. But they speculate that the kidney may be "immunologically privileged," thus allowing the transplanted cells to survive.

The attempt to transplant islet cells rather than the whole pancreas represents a growing trend in transplantation, from what might be called anatomic grafts to physiologic grafts. The aim in the latter case is to replace one, or a few, vital functions. If this can be achieved by transplanting a couple of syringefuls of donor cells, rather than an entire organ, this is, of course, easier — and is thus the preferred way.

The cells may be easier to obtain than a whole organ, as well as simpler to administer. More important, current technology allows transplanters to grow some cells in lab dishes, multiplying their numbers, so that smaller amounts of donor cells may be needed from human donors. The cells also may be manipulable, so that immunologic incompatibilities that would lead to rejection can be erased. It may be possible, also, to form hybrid cells between the donor and host that perform the required physiologic function — produce insulin, for example — but are recognized as "self" by the recipient.

The most efficient such transplants — and the most useful — may not affect the large internal organs like the liver and heart. Rather, they may involve central control areas for these organs in the brain.

Some major body functions are being shown to be controlled from rather small, discrete areas in the brain. Replacement or supplementation of these control areas holds promise of therapeutic results.

This possibility is particularly exciting, researchers say, because some experiments indicate there is very little risk of immunologic rejection: Brain cells appear not to trigger rejection when transplanted into another brain. This suggests it even may be possible to use brain cells or tissues from nonhuman primates like chimpanzees for transplantation into humans. This could ease transplanters' difficulty in obtaining donor brain cells.

One of the first human brain cell transplants was conducted in the early 1980s by clinical researchers at the Karolinska Institute in Stockholm, Sweden. They were trying to correct the neurologic condition called Parkinson's disease, characterized by tremors, difficulty in walking, and other distressing symptoms.

The current belief is that Parkinson's disease occurs because the muscle control center in the brain, called the corpus striatum, receives too little of the chemical dopamine, which is a neurotransmitter. Dopamine helps carry the brain's orders to the muscles, to initiate voluntary movement. Without it, the muscles act out of control. Much of the dopamine used in the brain is produced by a group of cells near the brain stem, called the substantia nigra. In patients with Parkinson's disease, however, these cells seem to be defective or absent.

The Karolinska doctors attempted to compensate for this loss by transplanting pieces of adrenal gland, which also produces dopamine, into the brain. One of the two initial subjects appeared to regain some muscle control as a result. Neither patient appeared to suffer transplant rejection, or any of the other severe side effects that may follow transplant surgery. These results have encouraged the Swedish research team to continue their efforts. They currently are gearing up to transplant dopamine-producing cells from a human fetus into Parkinson's victims' brains, thereby raising another ethical issue: the use of fetal tissues, from abortions and stillborns, for medical treatments.

Heartened by the Swedes' results, neurosurgeon Ignacio Madrazo, of La Raza medical center in Mexico City, and several of his colleagues reported, in 1987, that they were performing autotransplants in which relatively large, intact pieces of one of a

Parkinson's patient's adrenal glands are transplanted, intact, into his or her brain. The transplanted tissue is clipped in place near the substantia nigra, where it is continually bathed in spinal fluid. The Mexicans reported, in the *New England Journal of Medicine,* that both of the patients on whom they performed this operation showed clear signs of clinical improvement — and they quickly operated on nine others. However, two of the eleven died within months of the surgery, for unknown reasons.

Neurosurgeons from the United States were deeply impressed by the Mexicans' results. "I think I have witnessed history!" a New York neurosurgeon, Dr. Abraham N. Lieberman, declared after visiting them. He predicted that the operation soon would be performed widely in the United States. In Nashville, at Vanderbilt University, the first American patient, Mrs. Dickye Baggett, told reporters a week after her self-transplant:

"I'm not shaking [from Parkinson's disease] at the moment. You do not know how grateful I am!"

Experiments in animals already have shown that many other patients, besides the victims of Parkinson's disease, may one day be helped by transplants into the brain. The severe, early form of senility that is called Alzheimer's disease, which destroys the lives of tens of millions of otherwise strong, healthy persons in their fifties and sixties, is believed to be caused by loss of cells that produce a neurochemical called acetylcholine. Transplants with acetylcholine-producing nerve cells already have been performed in monkeys. The hope is that similar transplants, in humans, will reverse the memory loss and confusion of Alzheimer's disease.

TRANSPLANTABLE TISSUES

The large, vital internal organs are not the only body parts that are now routinely taken from living or dead donors and transplanted into needy recipients. The other borrowed body parts often are characterized as tissue transplants. Tissues, which are the simpler subunits of organs, tend to be easier to recover, store, and use. Some can be kept indefinitely, until needed, in a dried or frozen state. Usually, too, a tissue transplant involves only a small portion of the donor's supply of that tissue, which the body can replace, unlike the whole organs, which it cannot.

Widely used tissue transplants include:

Corneas — The eye's clear window easily can be removed after death. Corneas can be preserved by freezing. When transplanted into persons whose corneas have been damaged, they improve vision in the large majority of cases. In the United States alone, 20,000 corneal transplants are performed each year. Eye banks to arrange these operations were started in the United States in the 1940s — and now exist in many other nations around the globe.

Blood — Although not often thought of in this way, a blood transfusion is a transplant. Indeed, it is a partial organ transplant, since many blood banks now regard blood, with its several different types of cells, as a liquid organ. The current practice is to divide whole blood donations into component parts — including red cells, plasma, platelets, and white cells — so that each donor can serve the particular medical need of several recipients.

Bone marrow — This tissue is transplanted in the attempt to bolster or re-create the immune system of persons stricken with lethal diseases such as leukemia and aplastic anemia. Heavy radiation destroys some marrow. After the nuclear reactor explosion at Chernobyl in the Soviet Union, more than a dozen Russians who were in or near the plant were given bone marrow transplants. A few survived who otherwise would almost certainly have died. The marrow includes cells that divide and multiply to form the white blood cells, which constitute a crucial part of the body's immunologic defenses. Marrow transplants have been difficult to develop because they often cause severe graft-versus-host disease, which threatens the recipient's life. Improved techniques, however, presage a widening medical role for them. Some 2,000 marrow transplants are performed in the United States each year. The marrow for these transplants usually is removed from living donors — often an immunologically close family member — by sucking it out of one of the pelvic bones through a needle while the donor is under anesthesia.

Skin — Burn patients, in particular, need covering to protect their wounds. Skin is the perfect human cover. Skin is obtainable from cadavers — and can be processed and stored for later use. In the United States, and probably in other countries as well, skin transplant material continues to be in very short supply. To overcome shortages, several groups of researchers are developing methods to grow skinlike membranes of human skin cells in the laboratory.

Bone — Hundreds of thousands of bone transplants are performed each year. The need arises when bones are shattered, become irreversibly infected, or are destroyed or removed surgically.

Overall, the transplant revolution in medicine has achieved its first major goals. The grafting of human kidneys, liver, heart, and pancreas is now an accepted — if difficult and expensive — tool of medical practice. Moreover, it is clear that experimental studies foretell far wider use of transplants. They are going to relieve many other serious and distressing medical conditions, as the twentieth century ends and the twenty-first century unfolds.

Chapter Five

Progress on Heart Disease

By Harry Schwartz

Harry Schwartz, a former editorial writer of The New York Times, *specializes in medical writing.*

"The health of the people is better than it has ever been before." This judgment, in these or similar words, has recurred frequently in official pronouncements by the government of the United States — under both Democratic and Republican presidents — during the past decade. The most impressive gains leading to this conclusion have been registered in the area of heart disease, despite the fact that now, as has been true for many years, more people in the United States die from cardiac ailments each year than from any other major cause of death. The fact that the number of older people is now rising far more rapidly than was ever expected earlier — greatly complicating financial and medical problems — is in large part related to the enormous progress that has been achieved against heart failure.

A few numbers relating to what has happened in the United States, where heart disease is particularly acute, will illustrate graphically not only the magnitude of what has been accomplished in conquering this killer but also the great dimensions of the task still remaining. In 1983, preliminary government data show, about 766,000 Americans died of heart disease, almost 40 percent of all deaths. Let us use 1960 as the baseline year against which to measure the progress that has been achieved. If the heart disease death rate in 1983 had been the same as in 1960, then the number of deaths in 1983 would have been 862,000, or almost 100,000 more than the actual number. This calculation reflects the fact that there were more people in this country in 1983 than in 1960. But another relevant fact is that the average age of the American population in 1983 was appreciably higher than it was in 1960, and, of course, the older a population, the more deaths we have to expect. If we take account of this aging of the American population by 1983, we find that in that year almost 1,295,000 people would have died of heart disease if no progress had been achieved since 1960.

It is the comparison between the 766,000 people who actually died of heart disease in 1983 and the almost 1,295,000 we would have expected to die of this cause if there had been no progress that points up the magnitude of the achievement here. Put most simply, in recent years only about 60 percent as many Americans have been dying annually of cardiac ailments as would have died — taking account both of the larger population and of the older population in this country — if this killer had remained as deadly as it was in 1960. White males, the largest group dying from heart disease, have obviously been great gainers from these advances, but so have all other significant groups in our population. And the gains have been spread through the age brackets, too, for heart disease claims victims from infants to the elderly.

One sign of the importance of this achievement is the fact that it has become the topic of an international discussion, particularly in such countries as Great Britain where little or no gain has been made in reducing heart disease death rates. Put most simply, the foreign debates can be summarized as "What are the Americans doing right that we aren't? What can we learn from the American experience that we can put to work in our own country so as to improve our own dismal record?"

The fact that there are such debates among able foreign

physicians and other scientists immediately indicates a central fact: Nobody in the United States can really explain exactly why the chance of dying of heart disease has been declining so rapidly there. The heart is a complex organ that is affected by numerous influences, some arising in each person's organism and others from the outside environment. As a result, heart disease is a multifactorial series of ailments about whose origin in any particular patient there is often great uncertainty. The decline of some types of heart disease is explicable, of course. Rheumatic heart disease, which used to be much more frequent than it is now, was normally the consequence of childhood infection that crippled the heart. The decline seems clearly related to the post–World War II availability of effective antibiotics, which cure most children's infections quickly and easily. But most heart disease is of other kinds, particularly coronary heart disease, whose diminution is not so easily explainable.

Another of the many current mysteries is why there is such a wide variation in the death rate from heart disease among different regions, variations that persist even after the data are corrected for the different age distributions in the various states. For example, in 1980, the age-adjusted death rates from heart disease for white males aged thirty-five to seventy-four varied from highs of 581 and 562 deaths per 100,000 population in West Virginia and Kentucky to lows of 322 and 324 deaths per 100,000 population in Hawaii and New Mexico. Similarly, among the analogous groups of white females, the highs were 237 and 217 deaths per 100,000 population in West Virginia and New York respectively to lows of 122 and 130 deaths per 100,000 population in Hawaii and New Mexico. Why are heart disease deaths so high in West Virginia and so low in Hawaii and New Mexico? For that matter, why are the male death rates so very much higher than the female death rates in the different states? We do not know.

The United States is obviously doing many things right with respect to heart disease, but just what it is doing right is the subject of the debate. One school of thought emphasizes life-style and claims most of the credit should be given to the changes in the way we live, in our nutrition, in how we play, and so on. The other major school of thought gives the major credit for saving so many lives to the enormous recent gains in medical knowledge and capabilities for treating heart disease. In this regard, too, it seems important that in the last two decades good medical treatment for serious illness has been available to the great majority of Americans regardless of income or race.

In all probability both sets of factors have been at work. On average, Americans probably have been living healthier lives, but for the millions who have become ill with heart disease, the availability of greatly improved medical treatment has undoubtedly been very important. We shall attempt here to explain the great progress made against heart disease deaths by exploring both sets of changes.

For each of us the continuance of life requires that from minute to minute all our tissues and cells are bathed in a constant flow of blood, which brings oxygen and nutrients and takes away carbon dioxide and other waste products. This continuous circulation requires the ceaseless beating of a most remarkable pump, the heart, which beats from sixty to one hundred times a minute, about 40 million times a year and about 3 billion times in an average life span. The heart pumps a total of about five quarts of blood a minute through the body, a total of almost 20 million barrels during a normal lifetime. Absolutely essential is the interaction between the heart and the lungs. The body's system of veins brings used, oxygen-deficient blood to the heart, which sends that blood first to the lungs — where waste carbon dioxide is exchanged for essential oxygen — and then sends the newly oxygenated blood to every cell in the body through the arteries and capillaries.

Weighing less than a pound in most people, the heart achieves its amazing, long-lived reliability through its simple but masterly construction. It consists of four chambers, the right atrium and the left atrium on top and the right and left ventricles on the bottom. Strictly speaking, the heart consists of two pumps, one composed of the right atrium and right ventricle and the other of the left atrium and left ventricle. But the beating of these two pumps is so well coordinated that we are justifed in regarding the heart as one single pump — at least so long as the rhythm of the heartbeats continues in its normal coordinated fashion.

In operation, used blood rich in carbon dioxide enters the right atrium, the reservoir from which it then goes to the right ventricle, whose rhythmic beat then sends this venous blood to the lungs where the essential exchange of oxygen for carbon dioxide takes place. The oxygenated blood then goes via the pulmonary veins to the left atrium and then to the left ventricle, from which a powerful contraction sends it through the aorta to the rest of the body. The right ventricle has a comparatively weak beat since it sends blood only the short distance to the lungs; the left ventricle's contractions account for about 80 percent of the total power of the heart, power required to send the revitalized blood to every cell in the body from the brain to the toes.

The power for the beating heart comes from that remarkable tissue, the enormously energetic heart muscle, or myocardium, which contracts and relaxes at least once every second through a lifetime, which may stretch to eighty, ninety, or even over a hundred years. Injury to the myocardium — in particular, death to any portion of it — poses the greatest danger to a continuance of the affected person's life. Such injury takes place most often when there is an interruption in the heart's own blood supply that brings oxygen and nutrition to the hardworking myocardium. The heart's blood supply makes its way through the essential coronary arteries that wind their way around the heart. The enormous amount of work done steadily by the myocardium is reflected in that muscle's ravenous need for oxygen brought by the blood. The myocardium uses 80 percent of the oxygen the coronary arteries bring it, a far higher percentage of the available oxygen supply than is used by any other organ. The regular beat of the heart is governed by the sinoatrial node, a tiny cluster of nerve cells in the rear wall of the atrium, which generates the weak electrical spark that sets off each round of muscle contraction and relaxation. Essential, too, are the four cardiac valves — one in each of the heart's four chambers — which control the flow of blood.

No man-made machine using even our most advanced technology can compete in reliability, durability, or complexity with the heart, whose total size is about that of an average adult's fist. But the facts that over 750,000 Americans die annually of heart disease and an estimated five and a half million Americans suffer from heart disease at any given time testify that hearts do break down and malfunction.

The most dramatic malfunction is the heart attack, which may kill quickly at any time and any place, or which may cripple the victim and make him or her subject to death days, weeks, or months later. A heart attack may be caused by a disastrous break in the even beat and its replacement by a chaotic fluttering, or fibrillation, that may soon end in complete cessation of all beats, or death. Or a heart attack may be caused by a sudden interruption of the coronary blood flow to the myocardium, an interruption that is soon followed by the death of more and more cells unless something can be done quickly to restore the blood supply to all or most of the heart muscle. The two catastrophes are not mutually independent, since any death of heart muscle will tend to end the even, healthy beat and replace it by an irregularity that worsens as the damage to the myocardium increases.

Either type of damage to the heart described above need not be immediately life threatening since there are gradations both in problems of the heartbeat and in the amount of damage to the heart muscle. The heart may run too fast — tachycardia — or too slow — bradycardia — for a wide variety of reasons without being immediately life threatening. Similarly, a person may have a myocardial infarction — the death of a portion of the heart muscle — which can be compensated for and which may reflect only a partial blockage of the coronary blood supply. But the heart is such a vital organ that no malfunction in its operation can be taken lightly.

There are mechanical problems that can arise in the heart. The valves between the atria and the ventricles and between the ventricles and the major blood vessels must fit tightly. If they don't, they leak and permit damaging backflow of the blood, a phenomenon that seriously damages the efficiency of the heart and increases the strain upon the myocardium. Such damage to the valves is a frequent consequence of childhood rheumatic fever. The amount of work the heart must do in pumping blood through the body depends upon the size of each individual, one reason why obesity can be dangerous to cardiac health. Finally, the amount of work the heart must do also depends upon the condition of the blood system. Are the arteries and veins smooth, so the blood flows with a minimum of friction, or are many of the blood vessels blocked by deposits of debris, the so-called atherosclerotic plaques, which narrow the channels and make it much harder for the heart to pump the requisite amount of blood throughout the body?

Some babies are born with deformed hearts that cannot do their work properly. Somehow the genetic instructions governing these babies' development in their mothers' wombs went awry, and the hearts these infants are born with are structurally very different from normal hearts. Until the past few decades these babies were doomed to die more or less quickly, since their hearts simply could not do the work required as these children grew older and larger. One of the great contributions of cardiac surgery since 1950 has been its ever-increasing ability to operate to change the internal structure of malformed hearts so that, often, the children involved have been able to grow up and live normally. In late 1984 the transplants of both human and animal hearts were made in infants, suggesting that ultimately babies with even the most defective natural hearts may be saved.

Finally, the heart is subject to the same enemy attacks as the rest of the body. Bacteria, viruses, and parasites may cause infection and inflammation of the heart muscle, damaging its work capacity, or the heart may develop cancer, though that is fortunately rare. Most mysterious of all the heart diseases are the cardiomyopathies, in which the myocardium degenerates and ceases to function properly, often for reasons no one knows or can do anything about.

We could list the large number of things that can go wrong with the heart or its functioning. But the remarkable fact is that for most human beings, this tiny, complex bundle of tissues does its job day after day, year after year, for many decades. Nevertheless, in the industrialized countries of the world and increasingly even in many developing countries, the major cause of heart disease is atherosclerosis, which progressively blocks the coronary arteries and, by reducing blood flow through the myocardium, threatens the continued health and functioning of this great heart muscle. Some degree of atherosclerosis may exist even in young people, but its prevalence and seriousness tend to increase with age.

Typically, atherosclerosis begins with some injury to the smooth lining of an artery, an injury that platelets — important in blood coagulation — cover and protect while the area is repaired. But in atherosclerosis, cells from the middle of the artery wall rise to the surface and infiltrate the wound. The result is an atheroma, a deposit of fats and fibers that at best leaves a bump, narrowing the affected artery. The worse the atherosclerosis, the more such deposits there are, the thicker and less elastic the artery wall becomes, and the more the lumen, or channel, narrows. The atherosclerosis may help precipitate a heart attack by aiding in the creation of a blood clot, which blocks the coronary artery entirely, or it may encourage an arterial spasm, which can also stop the flow of blood.

Anginal pain in the chest is a frequent early warning that coronary blood channels are narrowing and the myocardium is not getting enough oxygen to meet its needs. In a heart attack, the pain may be extreme, usually in the chest, but sometimes radiating to the arms or even to the stomach, where it can be confused with indigestion. Or the pain may be in the back, the jaw, or the neck. Frequently there is weakness, nausea, sweating, vomiting, great restlessness, and anxiety. But a myocardial infarction may be without pain initially, with the first signs being breathlessness, confusion, or a sudden drop in blood pressure. The development of the symptoms of a heart attack testify that the efforts to prevent such a disaster have failed and the victim needs the best resources of modern therapy. So let us look now first at what is generally known and believed about prevention of heart disease through life-style changes, and then at what medical knowledge and technology have to contribute toward preventing heart ailments and then treating them and their consequences if they occur.

Anyone who has watched the progress since the 1960s knows that a revolution has taken place in many areas of the world in life-style, a revolution intimately tied to a new preoccupation with maintaining health. People are smoking less, eating fewer saturated fats, watching their salt intake, and exercising more. Joggers have become a feature of the scene almost everywhere, while the crowds on the tennis courts and the golf courses seem to increase steadily. Some more exact data on these changes are given in this statement by Dr. Robert I. Levy of Columbia University, former head of the National Heart and Lung Institute at the National Institutes of Health:

"The consumption of cigarettes has changed markedly and the number of cigarette smokers has fallen. Since 1963, the consumption of tobacco has declined by over 29 percent. The consumption of fluid milk and cream is down over 22 percent, butter by over 36 percent, eggs by over 14 percent in this period. The consumption of saturated fats (fats of animal origin) and oils is down by over 48 percent, while the consumption of vegetable fats is up by 74 percent. The average American cholesterol intake, which used to be quoted at 600 to 800 milligrams per day, is now less than 500 milligrams of cholesterol per day."

But changes of life-style, it should be underlined, can only decrease the probability of heart disease, not guarantee that it will not happen. Even some assiduous joggers drop dead of a heart attack while running, as did famed runner Jim Fixx not long ago. Some cigarette smokers live happily into their eighties and nineties, becoming victims to neither lung cancer nor heart disease despite the statistical evidence of their high risk.

The point was probably best stated a few years ago by Dr. Fritz L. Meijler, a noted Dutch cardiologist, when he pointed out that while life-style changes in a large population improve matters for many people, "there is still no individual who can prevent his heart disease. One may give up smoking, one may change one's diet, one may lose weight and/or lower one's blood pressure, but still there is no guarantee that one will not be disabled by or die from coronary heart disease before the age of sixty." In short, we all live and die on the basis of probabilities whose exact application to each of us we cannot know in advance.

At the root of the problem is the fact that we do not yet know what complex of factors produces atherosclerosis in individuals. Certainly the evidence is great that cigarette smoking is involved, and that regular energetic exercise is good for most individuals. But genetics and our inherited traits are also involved, and each of us has a different heritage from our parents. The complexity of the problem is nowhere better illustrated than in the debate over cholesterol, the fatty substance that all those who minimize their intake of animal fats are trying to limit. In the spring of 1984 a major study was released indicating that patients who started with an excessive body load of cholesterol suffered less heart illness and death if they lowered their blood cholesterol by diet and by use of a drug that drains cholesterol from the body. On the basis of this report, many of the popular media trumpeted that the case had been proved, that cholesterol was the "villain" causing heart disease and heart disease deaths. But in the medical community, the controversy continued. The study had concentrated on people who started out with a heavy load of cholesterol, so what relevance did it have to the great majority of people who don't have that problem (hypercholesterolemia, in medical jargon)? asked the skeptics. Moreover, cholesterol is manufactured in the bodies of healthy human beings, since it is an essential constituent of certain vital organs. Hence the debate goes on about what contribution, if any, high consumption of cholesterol-containing foods makes to promoting coronary heart disease. The balance of informed opinion seems to be that it is wise to cut down on foods containing saturated fats, particularly if one has a high blood cholesterol level, and it is this preponderance of expert opinion that most Americans seem to have accepted in changing their diets in the past twenty-five years.

Major economic as well as health issues rest on these debates. Dairy farmers, cattle growers, and egg producers are bitter because their markets have been cut by what they regard as "unjustified propaganda" against their products. On the other hand, the fishing industry has seen demand for its products rise as people have learned that fish are low in cholesterol, though that is not true of other foods from the sea, such as shrimp and lobster.

Further complicating the debate is the fact that the fats in our blood have been fractionated and analyzed so that now the real enthusiasts in this field speak of high density lipoproteins (HDL, good) and low density lipoproteins (LDL, bad), and it is to these we are now told to look to divine our risks of heart disease.

Stress is another factor that has been popularly tagged with responsibility for heart disease. Some doctors have written of Type A individuals as being at special risk of heart attacks. A Type A individual is stereotyped as the ambitious, achieving person who seeks never to waste a minute, is typically doing ten things more or less simultaneously, and who constantly feels the heavy weight of obligations. But here again there are mysteries. True, top business executives are sometimes killed by premature heart attacks, but many go on for years with fantastically heavy schedules. And some studies show that top executives don't necessarily die any younger than other individuals with fewer responsibilities and smaller incomes. Moreover, the skeptics can point to individuals such as President Reagan, Armand Hammer, the head of Occidental Petroleum, and Leon Hess, the head of Amerada Hess, as examples of elderly individuals who have coped and continue to cope with loads of stress far beyond the average. Winston Churchill is, of course, the most famous example of one who violated all the rules. He lived into his nineties despite his heavy responsibilities as Britain's leader during World War II, and his personal habits included smoking many cigars every day and drinking a reported quart of brandy daily for many years.

But after all the debate and the uncertainties and the probabilities have been taken into account, it seems most unlikely that the major changes in American life-style since 1960 and the improvements in the cardiac health of the American people are unrelated. On the contrary, it seems much more likely that the changes away from cigarette smoking, toward lower-fat diets, toward more active lives, and toward at least moderation of stress have helped many people. But these changes in life-style have not been universal panaceas and are unlikely ever to become such.

We turn now to the role of medical knowledge and technology in helping to avoid heart disease and to treat these ailments most effectively when they do strike.

In the sphere of prevention there is no doubt about the most important accomplishment, the effective attack on high blood pressure (hypertension), which is universally agreed to be a major cause of heart disease. The recognition of the importance of high blood pressure was the first major step because it stimulated energetic action more than a decade ago to identify victims and to help them cope. Because blood pressure is measured on a continuum, the limits defining high and low blood pressure are necessarily always somewhat arbitrary. Moreover, the limits of "normal" also tend to change with increasing age, further complicating the issue. Blood pressure, as many people know, is measured by two numbers: one, the systolic pressure, is the highest level registered during one heartbeat; the other, the diastolic pressure, is the lowest level registered during one heart beat. A person whose blood pressure is, say, 120/80 will be congratulated by his or her physician. Someone whose blood pressure is 210/120 will be regarded as very sick and may even be hospitalized. A blood pressure of, say, 140/90 falls in a debatable range where some physicians would feel treatment to reduce the pressure was desirable, while others would question the need.

How can blood pressure be reduced? In some people, though by no means all, the reduction can be obtained by cutting down salt intake. Others can do it by changing their diet, losing weight, or even by engaging in some kind of meditation or quiet periods daily. But for most people the surest and most effective way of reducing blood pressure is by using one or several drugs of the vast armamentarium now available. Diuretics, which increase one's excretion of water, are often used, and they tend to reduce blood volume. Other drugs lower blood pressure by dilating the blood vessels, providing more space through which the same amount of blood courses. Still others slow the heartbeat, thus reducing the volume of blood passing through the arteries in a given time period. Some patients can be helped easily with a single drug. Others have blood pressure that defies even three or four usually effective drugs used concurrently. Treatment, in short, must be individualized by one's doctor, who bears in mind the good to be done by lowering blood pressure but also seeks to avoid the harmful side effects that even the best medicines may have on some who take them.

Very impressive is the progress that has been made in alerting people to the problem of blood pressure and in motivating many who suffer from high blood pressure to undergo treatment. In 1972, 50 percent of all Americans with hypertension didn't even know they had the problem; now that percentage is below 20 percent. In 1972 only about one-eighth of all patients with high blood pressure, about 4 million people, were using effective therapy. The latter figure is now estimated to substantially exceed 10 million people. Some community surveys have indicated that as many as 90 percent of all hypertension victims now know of their problem and as many as half may be receiving treatment.

Diagnosis and therapy rather than prevention still comprise most of the work done by physicians, and in both of these areas vast advances have been made in recent years and continue to be made now. The old standbys — the stethoscope, the electrocardiogram, the chest X ray — still occupy their honorable and useful places in diagnosis and may be employed in a patient at rest or during a stress test. Heart disease can be looked for in a routine annual physical examination or it can be suspected if the patient has symptoms — chest pain, breathlessness, a rapid heartbeat, and so on — that suggest there are problems with the vital pump that keeps each of us alive.

The physician who suspects heart trouble after the usual superficial examination now has a wealth of techniques available to help decide if there is something wrong, and, if there is, to help pinpoint the exact nature of the problem and its location in the heart. Let us remember that the heart is a complex organ and problems may arise in the myocardium, in the coronary arteries, in the valves separating the different chambers, in the mechanism that controls the beat, as well as in hormones, neurotransmitters, and other influences acting upon the heart from the rest of the body. This multiplicity of possible problems has led to the development of numerous techniques for trying to study the heart and its malfunctioning.

Where possible, the physician will use a noninvasive technique, with an eye to causing the patient minimum trouble and danger. The patient may be asked to wear a Holter monitor, a device that measures and records on tape the pattern of the heartbeat over a long period so that the physician can spot the occasional malfunction that does not show up in an ordinary electrocardiogram taken during a few minutes. Or a radioactive isotope — thalium or technetium, usually — may be injected into the blood and then followed by means of radiation counters, which show the pattern of blood flow through and around the heart as revealed by the pattern of radioactivity recorded. Several different varieties of ultrasound can be used to bombard the heart with ultrasonic sound waves that, depending upon the method used, can show the structure of the beating heart or give evidence of how the heart is functioning in different ways.

But the most remarkable progress in noninvasive diagnosis of the heart will probably be realized in the years immediately ahead. For example, the Imatron Company is introducing a high-speed CAT scanner that will provide real-time X-ray movies of the beating heart, taking thirty to sixty pictures a second, and showing an anatomic picture of the heart and the blood going through it in detail never before possible. Then there are the magnetic resonance imaging (MRI) machines, which use radio waves and their impact upon the individual atoms of the heart to give a picture of the physiology of heart functioning such as has never before been available. Finally, there is positron emission tomography (PET), which gives a view of the heart that adds still more detail and new dimensions.

These last machines will not be common everywhere until 1990 or later. For many years now, however, physicians have had an invasive method of studying the heart, which, while posing some small degree of risk, has added enormously to diagnostic capabilities. This technique is called angiography. It employs very thin flexible tubes — catheters — which are threaded through the arteries and veins until they reach the heart. Sometimes the catheters can be used to visualize the blockages in the coronary arteries or to measure blood pressure at key points inside the heart. Once the catheters are in place, they can be used as channels to introduce opaque dyes into the blood circulation, and those dyes can be followed by X rays to produce moving pictures of the heart's blood circulation and of trouble spots in that circulation.

Historically, coronary angiograms as described above have required that patients be hospitalized for three days, with all the cost that implies. Recently a new machine has been introduced that permits such coronary angiography to be done on an outpatient basis, cutting the time needed to three hours. Essentially this new machine marries the computer to the X-ray movie camera. By using the computer to enhance the images received, physicians can use much less dye than in the conventional technique and also employ narrow tubes or catheters. Thus cost and time are reduced while the essential information is gathered so a decision can be made whether or not to operate on a patient.

We now assume that the patient's physician has made a diagnosis. The patient does have a variety of heart disease. What can be done about it?

The answer depends upon what is wrong and, as we indicated above, many things can go wrong with the heart; therefore, there are many possible therapies.

To look at the most dramatic case first, a man or woman has collapsed or is in intense pain because of a heart attack. In some cities, like Seattle, much of the population has been trained in cardiopulmonary resuscitation (CPR). In these communities, the chances are good that if an individual collapses a bystander can begin the process of trying to keep the victim's lungs working and blood receiving oxygen by giving mouth-to-mouth resuscitation and by manipulating the chest in an effort to get the heart beating again in a rhythmic fashion. Meanwhile the word has gone out for the paramedics, who, if they arrive in time, can use a defibrillator, an electrical device, to restart a heart that has halted or to put a heart that is in chaotic arrhythmia into the even, regular sinus beat that is essential for good cardiac health.

Once a heart attack victim is in the hospital, he or she can be put into the coronary intensive care unit, where highly trained nurses keep watch twenty-four hours a day. The patients in such a unit have their electrocardiograms, their pulses, and other vital functions monitored continuously. If they show signs of going into cardiac arrhythmia, the defibrillator is ready to shock their heart back into an even beat. And even before this emergency, the patient has received antiarrhythmia drugs, which tend to fight the forces making the heart's electrical system stop its even regular beat. A Swann-Ganz catheter monitors arterial pressure and left ventricular filling pressure to guard against the failure of the heart's basic pumping power. One hundred percent oxygen is often supplied to assure maximum oxygenation of the blood, while drugs to increase the blood pressure may be given so as to augment the sick heart's deficient work capacity. Morphine or other painkillers are given to relieve the excruciating angina often suffered by heart attack victims. In short, everything possible is done in a cardiac intensive care unit to counteract the deadly heart failure of the original heart attack. The result: more people survive heart attacks than used to survive in the days when there was no treatment but rest. Yet the cost of the close attention given in a cardiac intensive care unit is high, and some question whether every possible victim should receive this help.

Since a heart attack is often precipitated by the formation of a clot that completely closes off a coronary artery already narrowed by atherosclerosis, the closure cutting off blood and oxygen from the heart muscle brings on the threat of immediate death. So why not try to enter the coronary artery and somehow or other remove the impediment and restore the blood flow before it is too late? Cardiac surgeons had earlier thought of that possibility, but the question was always how.

Now such procedures are being done; heart attack victims are being operated on within a few hours after their attacks to reverse the stoppage in the coronary artery or arteries. Again, the key instruments are the thin tubes, or catheters, described above. Once these tubes are in place, doctors now may instill one of two drugs, urokinase or streptokinase, to dissolve the clot and open the channel so blood can flow again. Other techniques are being worked on, too. Instead of streptokinase or urokinase, some doctors have begun working with a product of biotechnology, tissue plasminogen activator, which some believe is more effective in dissolving clots. Some doctors are experimenting with lasers to blast away the obstructions hindering blood flow in the victim's arteries. In short, the trend is now toward more active intervention to reverse a heart attack, not merely to give the patient the best passive care in the hope that the patient's own body can summon up the reserves needed to survive.

Many patients now undergo heart operations that they hope will improve the quality of their lives and perhaps prevent a heart attack. These are the coronary artery bypasses, which were first introduced a decade and a half ago. Perhaps 175,000 of these operations are being done annually, and as many as a million of them may have been performed in this country since they were first introduced. The motivation for the patient to undergo the risks, discomfort, and expense of this operation is usually serious anginal chest pain, which may disable the victim and prevent him or her from living a normal life or just even enjoying life.

In the coronary artery bypass, near blockages in the coronary arteries are identified through coronary angiography as described above. Then the surgeon opens the patient's chest and literally provides new channels for the coronary blood to bypass the areas where obstructions have built up. The bypasses are strips of vein from the leg that are attached to the affected coronary arteries before and after the obstructions so that the blood may continue to flow as freely as possible. As many as a half-dozen bypasses may be provided for a single patient, depending upon the situation. The operation is complex, and therefore expensive, and not without risk. But for the great majority of patients who have it, anginal pain disappears completely or mostly, and for patients who have a particularly serious type of heart disease, this operation extends life by years. Moreover, in the best medical centers the risks of this operation are small.

The ability to do this complex procedure successfully has obviously resulted from a long process of development. The key contribution here has been the development of the heart-lung machine, an artificial pump and oxygenator through which the patient's own blood is circulated and provided with oxygen while the operation is in progress. With the heart-lung machine doing the necessary pumping and oxygenation of the blood, the patient's own heart can be stopped and worked on carefully. The ability to see the heart and to have it fully quiet is vital in this operation as the surgeon performs the exquisitely delicate cutting and sewing that are the essence of putting in the desired bypasses. Then when the operation is finished, the blood vessels are connected again to the reconstructed heart, which begins beating evenly under the impetus of an electric shock.

Progress is incessant in modern cardiology, where many ingenious minds and skillful hands labor to help sick people. Why should it be necessary to open the chest, stop the heart, and perform this reconstructive surgery? Can't the obstructed coronary arteries be cleaned directly so as to restore or improve blood flow through them? These are the questions some doctors asked as the flood of coronary bypass operations grew and grew. The result of this questioning has been the development of what is known as angioplasty, a technique in which the coronary arteries are invaded directly to improve the blood flow. Angioplasty is a further extension of angiography. Here catheters, thin tubes, are introduced into the coronary arteries and followed through X-ray monitoring. These tubes contain balloons at their ends, and when a catheter reaches an obstruction, the balloon is inflated and pressed against the obstruction. The result is frequently to depress the height of the atherosclerotic mound and thus to increase the diameter of the channel through which the blood flows, a direct solution to the same problem the surgeon attempts to solve with bypasses. Angioplasty is quicker and cheaper, and the patient avoids the risks of having his chest opened and his heart stopped. But angioplasty can itself precipitate a heart attack, so it is sometimes done with a cardiac surgeon, his team of helpers, and the needed equipment available on a standby basis to take over if catastrophe strikes.

But even angioplasty requires that the body be invaded with catheters and bombarded with X rays, all of which carry some risk. Hence the interest in the claim of many cardiologists that some fraction of the patients treated with coronary artery bypass operations or angioplasty can be equally well treated simply by medicines alone. This assertion is not made for all patients for whom operations are recommended but for perhaps 10 to 20 percent, 25,000 or so annually.

The key to this belief that many more patients with serious heart obstructions can be managed without operations of any kind is the fact that the number, variety, and capabilities of drugs to treat heart conditions have grown remarkably since the early

1960s. Digitalis has been used by doctors for about 200 years to strengthen the heart's pumping action so it can cope with its load. Nitroglycerin tablets began being used a century ago to help patients relieve the pain of sudden, sharp anginal attacks. Diuretics, discovered early in the period after World War II, rid the body of surplus water, thus reducing the volume of blood an overworked heart must pump.

A group of remarkable modern drugs — the beta blockers, the calcium channel blockers, the angiotensin-converting enzyme (ACE) inhibitors, and others — now give doctors unprecedented powers to affect the operation of the heart, and in particular to ease the burden on a damaged or weakened heart. Most important from the patient's point of view is the fact that some of the newer drugs are superior to nitroglycerin and nitrate drugs in ending or at least moderating the pain of angina. That pain normally arises as a sign that the heart muscle, or myocardium, needs more oxygen and nutrition to do its work. It is precisely the excruciating pain of severe angina that sends many patients to the cardiac surgeons for a coronary artery bypass. So there is clearly competition between medical therapy and surgical therapy, both of which can often relieve or end the pain of angina and thus make the patient more comfortable and less fearful. Where medicine does not work, of course, the patient is more likely to become interested in a bypass operation or in angioplasty to relieve discomfort and fear.

The beta blockers are outstanding among drugs that can help relieve or end anginal pain. They are medicines which exert their influence on a group of specialized body cells that, among other functions, receive instructions from the brain calling upon the heart to increase its beat or upon the veins to constrict in response to perceived emergencies or stresses. Either of these responses would make an injured heart's work more difficult, increase the myocardium's need for oxygen and nutrition, and thus presumably increase the anginal pain. What the beta blockers do is prevent these cells — the so-called beta receptors — from responding to the brain's instructions. Or, put another way, the beta blockers tend to slow the heartbeat and to dilate or widen the veins. By easing the work load on the heart, the beta blockers reduce the myocardium's need for oxygen and therefore tend to relieve anginal pain when it occurs. The beta blockers and other new drugs can also keep the heart in proper rhythm, blocking the forces that tend to make the heart beat too fast. Other available drugs permit physicians to make similar and other useful adjustments to the heart's functioning and to the environment of the blood system so as to ease the load on the heart.

A sad part of the history of these drugs, particularly the beta blockers and the calcium antagonists, is that the United States was very late in permitting them to be used by American physicians. They were not allowed on the market here until many years after they were being used routinely in Japan, Western Europe, and much of the rest of the world. The Food and Drug Administration (FDA) said it was not approving these drugs because it had questions about their safety. Those who supported the FDA's delays seemed never to consider the benefits these medicines could give to patients, benefits that were denied so long as these drugs were not approved for use by American physicians. It is perhaps a coincidence, but the steep decline in United States heart disease mortality began about the same time the FDA approved the first beta blocker, and that decline has continued in the intervening years during which the FDA has adopted a more permissive attitude toward letting American doctors use new drugs to treat heart disease. (It must be recorded that for years British medical magazines routinely told their readers not to pay any attention to American books on cardiology, asserting that those books could not recommend really modern therapies because many of the essential heart drugs had not been approved by the FDA and thus were denied American physicians.)

Ironically, the U.S. government, whose agency, the FDA, did so much to block the use of modern heart drugs for years, has more recently helped discover and verify one of the most important uses of some of these drugs. The National Heart, Lung and Blood Institute several years ago sponsored an extensive clinical test — involving thousands of patients — to see whether a beta blocker could, as many doctors believed, lower the rate of deaths in people who had had heart attacks. In 1981 the institute called off its clinical test prematurely because it had become so clear that the beta blocker was saving lives that it was deemed unethical to deny the control patients in the test the help that drug could give them. Yet fifteen years earlier, an influential group of officials in the FDA had sought to keep beta blockers off the American market on the basis of what is now recognized as an incorrect claim that beta blockers caused cancer.

Before we conclude this section, a few words are justified about the calcium channel blockers, or calcium antagonists. These have excited special attention in recent years as cardiologists have become aware that one cause of blockage in the coronary arteries may be arterial spasm. Calcium is one of the elements necessary to produce an arterial spasm in the first place, so the calcium antagonists, by blocking the flow of calcium to the relevant nerves, make arterial spasm less likely. These drugs also tend to dilate arteries, making it easier for a weakened heart to pump blood through a patient's circulatory system.

As a commentary on the effectiveness of cardiac drugs for helping patients, it is worth noting that the great Alabama football coach, Bear Bryant, who died earlier this decade, led his team through three of the greatest seasons of his career while seriously ill with heart disease. His condition was not revealed until after his death, when it became known that he had performed prodigies of team training and direction while taking different cardiac drugs prescribed by his doctors, drugs that permitted him to continue functioning despite his severe illness. On the other hand, proponents of coronary artery bypass surgery can point to a whole galaxy of eminent figures who have been helped by this procedure, including such well-known and active people as Henry Kissinger, the author Arthur Hailey, and many others.

The ability of surgeons to help disease victims is not limited to coronary artery bypass procedures. Every year hundreds of thousands of people, for example, have pacemakers inserted in their chests to regulate their heartbeat, usually to guard against bradycardia, a condition in which the heart beats too slowly and thus does not provide enough oxygen to the body. Pacemakers, which once were crude, large devices powered by electricity, which had to be obtained from a plug inserted into a wall socket, are now very small. They have their own tiny long-lasting batteries, so that the wearer of a pacemaker can go anywhere or do anything desired. The complex modern pacemaker can radio reports on its functioning and on the functioning of the heart of its wearer so as to inform the patient's cardiologist about what is going on. The cardiologist, from a distance, can also change the settings of the pacemaker so as to speed up or slow the heartbeat, as appropriate. The late Soviet leader Leonid Brezhnev wore a pacemaker in the last period of his life, and so does former West German Chancellor Helmut Schmidt. It is estimated that over half a million Americans now wear pacemakers.

As this is being written, it is expected that shortly several companies will introduce a new pacemaker with capabilities far exceeding those now on the market. The new pacemakers, it is reported, will also have the capability of giving the heart of the individual involved an electrical shock to restart that heart if it has stopped or to restore even sinus rhythm if the heart has gone into chaotic beating or fibrillation. Such a device, if widely available, might save thousands of people annually who now die suddenly because their hearts stop or go into a chaotic pattern of beats and then stop before paramedics equipped with a defibrillator arrive on the scene.

The insertion of a pacemaker is a relatively simple operation and does not require that the heart be stopped and the blood be passed through a heart-lung machine. But another procedure that does require open heart surgery, and hence use of the heart-lung machine, is a valve replacement operation, which becomes necessary when one or more of the four heart valves does not operate properly, either because of injury from infection or because of mechanical damage. One frequent result of malfunctioning of the valves is congestive heart failure. In this condition excess water accumulates in the lungs, and eventually unfortunate patients can literally drown in their own body fluids. The excess water accumulates because a valve defect impedes the flow of blood and prevents the heart from pumping enough blood so that the kidneys can remove the full amount of waste water needed to keep the body in a healthy state.

Three kinds of replacement valves are available for patients who need them. There are mechanical valves, usually made of plastic. Alternatively, valves may be transplanted from a dead human being or, more often, from an animal such as a pig. Because they are made of cartilage rather than soft tissue, human or animal valves do not pose the possible rejection problems faced in other kinds of transplants. Whichever valve is used, a successful operation of this kind can literally cure this kind of congestive heart failure.

We turn now to the most dramatic chapter of cardiac medicine, the developing capability of heart surgeons to replace an entire heart that is no longer capable of performing its work. As this is being written, there has been experience with three kinds of replacement hearts: human, animal, and artificial.

The most frequent procedure has been transplantation of a human heart from a person who is brain dead to another person who is well except for a seriously defective heart. This procedure began with the historic first transplant done by South African surgeon Christiaan Barnard almost two decades ago. This volume contains a chapter on transplants, so we will only summarize the story here. Most of the early wave of heart transplant patients at the beginning of the 1970s died fairly quickly because, fundamentally, of the inability of medicine at that time to deal with the rejection problem. In particular, if a patient was heavily medicated to overcome rejection, that patient was likely to die of infection because the means used to make rejection less likely weakened the entire set of body defenses against external invasion, and in particular against infection of any kind.

That problem has been considerably eased by a number of more recent developments, of which the discovery of a new drug, Sandimmun (cyclosporine), is the most important. Sandimmun permits the patient's body to fight rejection while leaving much of the immune system intact to fight infection. The result has been that many more heart transplant recipients are surviving for considerable periods of time, and the operation makes much more sense now than it did back in the early 1970s. The pioneers who have made much of this progress possible have been Dr. Norman Shumway and his colleagues at the Stanford University Medical Center, who stuck with heart transplants for many years despite many discouragements, and Dr. Jean Borel, the Swiss pharmacologist working for Sandoz Inc., who first identified cyclosporine as a potentially useful drug while screening fungal products found in samples of earth brought from Wisconsin and from Norway.

Xenotransplantation, the transplantation of an animal organ to a human being, was pioneered in the heart field by Dr. James Hardy of the University of Mississippi, who in 1964 transplanted an adult chimpanzee heart into a man of sixty-four. That patient lived only a few hours. Three later xenotransplants in Britain and South Africa also failed. But on October 26, 1984, physicians at Loma Linda University Medical Center in California transplanted a baboon heart into Baby Fae, an infant only a few days old and doomed to die because of a congenitally defective heart. The first few days of Baby Fae's life with the baboon heart provided pleasant surprises as the infant initially showed no signs of rejecting the baboon heart and was able to live even after all medical assist devices were removed. An important factor in this early success appears to have been the availability of Sandimmun, which seemed to have helped fight rejection of the baboon heart as effectively as it helps fight rejection of a transplanted human heart. Twenty days after the implantation, the infant's body did reject the heart and she died. Right up until just a few days before her death, however, the quality of her life was clearly better than it had been before the operation. Then she had desperately gasped for breath and struggled for every bit of nourishment. Even that temporary improvement meant to the Loma Linda doctors that, though much remains to be learned, animal-heart transplantation does hold promise.

Interest in using animal hearts for transplantation arises because of the extreme shortage of human hearts for the tens of thousands of people who could benefit each year from a new heart. The use of animal hearts has provoked sharp opposition, however, from animal-rights activists who had earlier exerted significant political pressure to curb even essential experimentation on animals to help learn more about means of curing human ailments. In any case, the economics of raising a primate such as a baboon to the point where its heart becomes useful for transplantation seemed to raise problems requiring further consideration.

The ideal solution could be the development of an artificial heart manufactured in the numbers required to meet the needs of all the people who must have new hearts to avoid death. It was this fact that evoked the huge wave of world interest in the case of Dr. Barney B. Clark, sixty-two years old, who received the first artificial heart transplant — a Jarvik-7 heart — in Salt Lake City in December 1982. Because of rules and obstacles hindering this first experiment, Dr. Clark did not receive his heart until he was almost dead. In particular, his lungs and other vital systems had been badly damaged by the nearly complete failure of his own natural heart. The result of this unfortunate situation was that Dr. Clark had a very difficult time with his artificial heart. Yet shortly before he died, 112 days after getting his artificial heart, Dr. Clark was shown on national television speaking briefly, but entirely rationally, with his surgeon, Dr. William DeVries.

To some people it appeared that this very expensive operation — in terms of the quarter-of-a-million-dollar hospital bill rolled up by Dr. Clark — had not been worth the return. A strong movement developed to prevent Dr. DeVries from implanting a second artificial heart at the University of Utah Medical Center. Obstruction from local opponents and also from the Food and Drug Administration finally so frustrated Dr. DeVries that he left Utah and shifted his base of operations to the Human Heart Institute International in Louisville, Kentucky, operated by the private Humana hospital chain.

There, Dr. DeVries attempted a second implantation, for a fifty-two-year-old former government employee who was on the verge of death from heart disease and who, because of his diabetes, was ineligible for human heart transplantation. William Schroeder was younger and generally healthier than Dr. Clarke had been, and seemed to make remarkable progress at first. He then suffered a series of strokes. Mr. Schroeder died after having lived 620 days with his Jarvik heart. Another patient, Murray Haydon, died after 488 days with this device in his chest. Still another patient, Jack

Burcham, died when the Jarvik heart proved to be too large to be contained in his chest cavity. A patient who received a Jarvik heart in Sweden had perhaps the best experience, living a relatively normal life with all his faculties for about six months, but then suffering a stroke and declining into death. As this is written, no Jarvik heart intended to be permanent has been implanted for almost two years, and much work is going on to improve the Jarvik heart — and also its potential competitors — so as to make blood clots and the strokes they bring less likely. Meanwhile, the Jarvik heart has been used successfully and repeatedly by surgeons who needed a "bridge," i.e., a means of keeping a desperately ill heart patient alive for a few days or weeks until a human heart could be found for transplantation.

Many of the opponents faced by Dr. DeVries seemed to think that the huge, ungainly apparatus used for Dr. Clark, for example, the 350 pounds of pumping equipment plugged to a wall electric outlet and carried on a golf cart, would always be essential to the artificial heart. They did not seem to understand that, like the first pacemaker, the first artificial heart was a crude device that would undergo very rapid improvement and miniaturization. Indeed, the prospects seemed reasonable for eventually doing away with the bulky equipment and replacing it with a much smaller device that could be carried in a shoulder bag for long periods of time. Ultimately, too, the artificial heart will no doubt be powered by batteries on a belt worn by the patient. Then the fact that a person has an artificial heart may be as little evident to the rest of the world as is now the fact that an individual has a pacemaker in his chest.

The ideal result is still some years away, but the whole history of rapid technological development in medicine makes such a happy outcome very likely. Already it is clear that the Jarvik heart, whether in its original or its improved form, will have competition, since several companies have been formed to try to develop alternative versions of an artificial heart. For example, a device called a left ventricular assist has been inserted in a California patient whose heart was failing after cardiac surgery. This device, essentially an additional pumping aid, is intended to help maintain the patient until a human heart can be obtained and transplanted into that patient, but the device could also be the basis for a future artificial heart. As mentioned above, the left ventricle of the heart supplies 80 percent of the heart's pumping power, which is why the left ventricular assist device was designed to help out when a patient's left ventricle cannot exert adequate power.

A more fundamental question has been raised by those who have qualms about the artificial heart. Can society afford this device? Many of the people who ask this question assume that either an artificial heart must be available to everybody or it should be available to nobody. This seems a harsh choice and is certainly not what exists today in the case of human heart transplantations, where the shortage of human hearts prevents everyone who needs one from getting it, although an ever-increasing number of these transplants (200 to 300 in 1984, for example) are being performed.

Some of those who question the economic feasibility of an artificial heart point out that more is involved than merely the fact that every year in the United States alone hundreds of thousands of people could benefit from having an artificial heart implanted in their chests. As we have seen, more than 750,000 people died of heart disease in 1983 alone. But estimates of the number of people suffering from heart disease now range around 5,500,000 and the number will undoubtedly rise as the United States population gets progressively older. Some observers suggest that if the artificial heart is truly successful, there will be a demand for prophylactic artificial heart insertions, i.e., the replacement of natural hearts that are still working but that have shown signs of weakness. And people who get one artificial heart may demand a replacement when their first shows signs of failing because of atherosclerosis or electrical malfunction or some other reason. Can our society afford to provide millions or tens of millions of Americans with artificial hearts, especially when most of the potential recipients would be elderly men and women, many of whom would be unlikely to work and pay taxes?

In essence, those who ask these questions are really asking how we would ration artificial hearts, assuming that they are developed and improved and become standard items of medical therapy as pacemakers and artificial heart valves are today. The rationing question is genuinely important, but it concerns only the question of who should benefit from a successful artificial heart. The problem here is reminiscent of the old Scottish recipe for rabbit stew that begins, "First catch your rabbit." Similarly, the first imperative is to encourage the further development and improvement of artificial hearts. As they become more available and are better able to help relieve human suffering and prevent premature death, our society will be able to debate and decide the rationing issues at its leisure.

As we look to the 1990s, the outlook for prevention, alleviation, and even cure of heart disease and associated ills such as heart attacks appears bright. In the area of drugs, two new approaches have roused much optimism. One was prompted by the discovery of atrial natriuretic factor (ANF), a hormone manufactured in the heart, which appears to have a powerful impact upon blood pressure. Much work is now going on to obtain this natural product in large quantity and to test it so that, if the hopes are correct, this hormone can be used as a drug to lower blood pressure. Then there is a new class of drugs of which the first on the market is likely to be one called lovastatin. These drugs apparently can reduce the low density lipoproteins and the very low density lipoproteins, which are now believed to be the components of cholesterol that do the damage in atherosclerosis. Additionally, the possibilities of dissolving atherosclerotic clots and thrombi in time to minimize the heart-destroying effects of a heart attack are looking up. Recent experiments with streptokinase have given a more optimistic view of its ability to dissolve blood clots without causing fatal hemorrhage elsewhere in the body. And probably sometime in 1987 or early 1988 the Food and Drug Administration will permit the marketing of tissue pasminogen activator, which some doctors believe will be the most effective means of dissolving coronary artery blockages that kill or maim so many people annually. But such techniques, based upon dissolving the coronary artery blockages, must be used within a very short time after a heart attack strikes. Meanwhile, work goes on to build better and cheaper artificial hearts, so that alternative cannot be dismissed despite the disappointing results of the first efforts to use Jarvik hearts as permanent replacements of human hearts. Heart transplants, now being done at the rate of over 1,000 a year, are increasing in number and in success. The chief restriction is the unfortunate fact that most suitable hearts are never donated for purposes of transplantation, but this situation is slowly changing as the need is more widely recognized. But in any case natural hearts can never satisfy more than a small fraction of the demand for new hearts to replace old, diseased ones.

In conclusion, the review above indicates not only that great progress has been made in reducing death from heart disease, but also that prospects are bright for further reducing such deaths. Ultimately, many cardiology researchers believe, we will learn the cause of atherosclerosis and be able to prevent or reverse it, thus eliminating the cause of most current heart disease. No one can tell how long it will take to obtain this essential knowledge. Meanwhile the fight to save heart disease victims with better drugs, new and improved medical devices (including artificial hearts), and an increased number of heart transplants (perhaps both human and animal hearts) will undoubtedly continue. Undoubtedly, too, Americans will increasingly try to prevent heart disease by changing their life-styles as more is learned about the factors that protect against this mass killer.

Chapter Six

Vaccines:
Triumph of an Age

By Harold M. Schmeck, Jr.

Harold M. Schmeck, Jr., who covers the biological sciences for The New York Times, *is the author of* The Semiartificial Man *and* Immunology: The Many-Edged Sword.

The child stared out at the world through wide, hopeless eyes set in a face all but obliterated by smallpox. Everywhere, from forehead to chin, a rough cobblestone pavement of crusts and sores had replaced the smooth skin of childhood.

This picture of a young smallpox patient, taken only a few years ago, is a part of history now. Mercifully, smallpox is no longer a fact of life anywhere on earth.

It was eliminated from the world's population by a prodigious decade-long effort that was probably the greatest single public-health triumph of the century.

The effort, costing many millions of dollars, was a remarkable feat of twentieth-century organization, logistics, and technology. But, in terms of medical science, it was almost as much a triumph

107

of the eighteenth as the twentieth century. The vaccinia virus, the active ingredient in smallpox vaccine, was probably a direct descendant of the cowpox virus that Dr. Edward Jenner used in 1796 when he introduced vaccination to the world and proved that it could prevent smallpox.

Indeed, the word *vaccination*, from the Latin word for cow, at first applied only to Dr. Jenner's preventive weapon against smallpox. For almost a century it was the only vaccine in existence. Almost a hundred years after Dr. Jenner's history-making experiment, the meaning of the word *vaccination* was broadened to include almost any kind of immunization. The change was suggested by Louis Pasteur, as a tribute to Jenner. Pasteur was himself a pioneer in vaccine research, having developed the first effective vaccine against rabies.

The smallpox virus will probably never again disfigure and kill humans, but vaccinia, the virus that conquered it, may well be put back into service soon to conquer other worldwide plagues that have always thwarted the forces of public health.

The idea of bringing vaccinia virus out of retirement, for uses that would have been inconceivable in Jenner's day, is one of a half-dozen or more new strategies that make public-health experts hopeful that a new age of vaccines is dawning that will have profound beneficial effects on human well-being throughout the world.

The future may hold new and much better vaccines against influenza, diphtheria, cholera, and other diseases. Vaccines have already been developed against one virus, that of hepatitis B, that is probably among the crucial causative factors in cancers that are all too common in the world.

Early human tests of two different malaria vaccines have already been made. They are a remarkable achievement considering the fact that, for centuries, the devastating disease was always considered beyond even the possibility of vaccine control.

By the mid-1980s a vaccine against AIDS, the deadly acquired immune deficiency syndrome, was also an urgently pursued goal, although few experts expected it to be brought to fruition soon.

Hardly any of mankind's other weapons against infectious

disease even approach vaccines in overall effectiveness. But many tragically widespread transmissible diseases of humans and animals have always been beyond their reach. Herpes viruses cause illness in over a million people in the United States alone. Often these infections are acquired through sexual intercourse and, in many cases, may contribute to cancer. No vaccine that is effective against herpes viruses exists today. Recently, papilloma viruses, related to those that cause warts, have at least partly replaced herpes viruses as cancer suspects. Vaccines against these viruses are lacking, too.

There are some regions of the world where fully one-quarter of all babies born alive die in their first year of life. Diarrhea, caused by bacteria and viruses, coupled with malnutrition and the debilitating effects of malaria and other parasite diseases, is responsible for this tragic death toll. Vaccines to deal with many of these infections are either nonexistent or are too expensive for the Third World.

By a paradox that may seen strange in the developed world, this frightful toll in babies' lives aggravates the world's greatest public-health problem — overpopulation. Parents who want a family and know that many of their babies are likely to die are not easily convinced that family planning makes any sense at all.

Vaccines might prevent much of this illness and death, but again, vaccines are either lacking or prohibitively expensive for nationwide use, particularly in the Third World.

Indeed, for impoverished regions of the world, even many of the vaccines that are taken for granted in the West are in tragically short supply. The World Health Organization, in 1987, said 2 million children are dying every year from measles, 600,000 die from whooping cough, and 800,000 die from neonatal tetanus. A quarter of a million children are affected by polio, and one in ten of them can be expected to die. Effective vaccines exist to protect against all of these. The World Health Organization is mounting a major campaign to have all the world's children protected against these diseases, and diphtheria and tuberculosis, too, where needed, by 1990.

In recent years, while all of these needs seemed to beckon so urgently, many vaccine manufacturers, particularly in the United

States, have been getting out of the business. Problems of liability made vaccine products difficult to justify on economic terms, and there seemed to be few really good new ideas for vaccine development. The swine flu program of 1976, in which more than 35 million Americans were immunized against a virus that never appeared, gave vaccines an undeserved bad name and further discouraged manufacturers.

But today there is a dramatically different outlook. Public-health experts speak of a dawning new era in vaccines and dare to hope that even worldwide diseases like malaria and hepatitis B may be conquered or at least controlled.

"Mankind is now on the threshold of a new era in the technology of vaccine development and production," said Dr. G. C. Schild and Dr. Fakhry Assaad of the World Health Organization. Their optimism stems from several new concepts for vaccine design, each made possible by advances in basic science.

In one such strategy, genes of flu viruses have been reassorted to make a harmless virus, which has a surface that appears to be identical to that of a flu virus that causes illness. This kind of benevolent trickery is the key to any live virus vaccine. The human immune system reacts defensively against the surface and stimulates immunity without illness. Conceptually, the trickery is a little like putting a slug in a subway turnstile, except, of course, that there is nothing dishonest about it.

Each particle of flu virus has eight genes packaged separately from each other. In the new vaccine, six come from a harmless laboratory version of the virus. The other two, giving the virus its surface profile, are borrowed from one that causes disease. Until the present, such manipulations of virus structure could be done only by indirect and imperfect means. Now the genes themselves are known quantities that can be manipulated almost at will. Scientists at the National Institutes of Health reported in 1984 that viruses with reassorted genes can indeed protect against influenza.

Unlike current flu vaccines, the new one is made from live, rather than inactivated, virus and is given by nose drops rather than injection. The nose-drop method is much more convenient for the patient and also gives a better quality of immunity against flu, some experts believe. The vaccine is undergoing large-scale tests.

Another strategy, on which pioneering work was done at the Research Institute of Scripps Clinic in California, goes even further. This strategy is to design and make vaccines from artificial chemicals. These are totally synthetic vaccines, a set of chemicals strung together in the laboratory to make a person's immune defense system think it has seen a whole virus. Having seen this mirage, the body builds immunity to it. In concept, this is a little like growing beefsteak from scratch in the laboratory without ever involving a cow in the process except for a few of its genes.

A third revolutionary idea is that of bringing vaccinia virus out of retirement for a whole new career — indeed, a new set of careers — by giving it new genes and therefore new identities that vaccinia virus never had before. To a virologist of a decade or so ago, this would be almost as startling as the idea of making wings of sparrows sprout from the backs of laboratory mice.

There are other new ideas as well, all based on discoveries in the esoteric science of molecular biology, particularly the techniques of recombinant DNA technology known as "gene-splicing."

Controversy has erupted over each of the new ideas. Each has its enthusiasts and its critics. There are also some people who would oppose all of the new strategies simply because they all involve recombinant DNA techniques. Some diehard opponents object to all aspects of gene-splicing work either as improper interference with the course of natural life or because they fear a new era of environmental pollution from the products of this new and potent biological technology.

Among all the new ideas for vaccine development, that of bringing vaccinia virus out of retirement is probably the strangest and one of the most controversial. Some scientists believe it may also be among the most promising of all.

It may also have an element of poetic justice. Vaccinia was the first and, by long odds, the most successful vaccine ever developed.

In the mid-1700s something called variolation was introduced from the Orient into British medical practice. It was simply the process of taking the crusts of smallpox sores from patients who survived mild cases of the disease and scratching this material into the skin of people who had not yet had smallpox. Sometimes these patients too got mild cases and were immune to smallpox thereafter. But also, more often than was reassuring, the person who had been variolated got a severe case of smallpox and died. The treatment was tolerated only because smallpox was such a fearful disease that risks were worth taking to combat it.

Vaccination began because Jenner noticed that people who milked cows often had a mild infection called cowpox, and that people who had experienced cowpox were always immune, thereafter, to the dread smallpox. Perhaps the equivalent of variolation could be done more safely with cowpox. In those days no one realized that the two diseases were caused by different viruses. No one knew what a virus really was. But the method worked, and the modern era of vaccination was born.

Doctors during the late 1700s and early 1800s did not actually prepare vaccine. Instead, they vaccinated one person from material from the sores of cowpox and then used the new vaccination sore as a source of material for the next recipients.

Vaccination was carried across the Atlantic to the New World by an even more bizarre method. Orphan children on their way from Europe to the Spanish colonies carried vaccinia by what amounted to a relay race of infection. The first child was infected with cowpox just before the ship sailed. The second was infected from the first child about eight days later; and so on all the way across the ocean. The voyage took many weeks, but there were many children and the last one who was inoculated still had a fresh cowpox sore, useful for further vaccinations, when the ship dropped anchor in the New World.

Like many developments in medicine, vaccination started out in fierce controversy. Cartoons in the British press showed people with the horned heads of cows growing out of their arms, implying that this was what came of vaccination. In those days, no one knew just what this material from cowpox was and many doubted that it was safe. Epidemics of smallpox continued while the controversy raged. Smallpox continued to erupt in the United States and many other developed countries for another 150 years.

But gradually, the evidence became too strong for even the most determined gainsayers. Where there was vaccination there simply was no smallpox.

What might have been the end of vaccinia's worldwide use came in 1977 when a ten-year global effort marshaled by the World Health Organization succeeded in eradicating smallpox. Today, the disease smallpox is only a tragic memory. The virus is still preserved in the freezer lockers of a few specially protected laboratories. So far as anyone knows, it exists nowhere else.

Smallpox vaccination as a routine public-health measure for civilians has all but disappeared. According to one expert, Albania is the only nation that still does it, immunizing its population against a disease that no longer exists because the memory of that dread disease still cannot be exorcised.

If the practice returns, it will be to conquer diseases other than smallpox. Dr. Bernard Moss and his colleagues at the National Institutes of Health and a research team led by Dr. Enzo Paoletti of the New York State Department of Health, independently of each other, have redesigned the vaccinia virus to produce an entirely new breed of live virus vaccine.

Vaccinia virus is by no means totally harmless. It can cause severe infection in patients who suffer from defects in their immune defense systems. For that reason, many specialists believe it should be used only against serious diseases. A prime candidate of this kind is AIDS, the acquired immune deficiency syndrome. It is a deadly virus disease for which no cure is available. By 1987 plans were being made to test the first experimental vaccines against AIDS. The use of vaccinia was one of the vaccine designs most seriously considered.

Retooled vaccinia viruses have already been used in experiments to protect mice against herpes viruses, chimpanzees against hepatitis B, and hamsters against flu viruses. The scientists believe this is only the beginning.

In order to understand how this is done, it is necessary to know a little about what a virus is and how it infects.

Viruses are strange particles that lie on the borderline between the realms of life and inert chemistry. The particles cannot quite be classed as living things. They cannot move, breathe, metabolize foods, or even reproduce by themselves, and thus they seem to be lifeless. Some viruses have actually been purified to the appearance of crystals. Once inside a living cell, however, a virus can reproduce. Its progeny emerge later as a whole new generation of virus particles.

The explanation is that viruses are really little more than packaged genes continually being cast about in the world until they find living cells to inhabit so that their genetic instructions can be put to work.

Vaccinia is one of the largest viruses known. It consists of an inner core of DNA (deoxyribonucleic acid), the active substance of the genes of all living things. The DNA of this virus is packaged in a globe-shaped coat of protein with spikes sticking out of it. When such a particle meets a living cell, the spikes make contact with matching structures on the cell surface. The virus becomes attached to the cell and invades it. In the process, the virus's load of DNA gets loose in the invaded cell. Thereafter, the genetic instructions carried in the virus's DNA subvert the cell's own genetic machinery and force it to manufacture a new crop of virus particles identical to the original one. When this has been done, the cell usually dies and the new crop of viruses break out to attack other nearby cells. All the effects that humans recognize as the symptoms of an infection are the results of cell damage and the reactions of the body's immune defense system to the invasion. The virus's core of nucleic acid carries the subversive message and does the main damage. But the identity of the virus, as the immune defenses see it, depends on the surrounding package. The structure of this package also determines what cells a virus is capable of infecting and which others it cannot penetrate. Only if a cell surface has something matching a part of the virus surface, like a key fitting into its lock, can the virus penetrate, release its genetic material, and set to work.

The new tools of recombinant DNA technology have made all of these things much more understandable than they were just a few years ago. Furthermore, the new techniques make it possible to take apart the genes of something like the vaccinia virus and to add or subtract new genetic messages almost at will.

That is how scientists are redesigning the vaccinia virus. They replace part of the virus's DNA with pieces of foreign DNA. The extra nucleic acid transplanted into the vaccinia virus carries instructions for making a substance that normally lies on the surface of another kind of virus and gives it its immunological identity.

When the hybrid viruses are made by the infected cell, each new particle will carry on its surface the identifying piece of the other virus, and the body will manufacture protective antibodies against it.

For example, Dr. Moss and his co-workers have put genes for the surface of the hepatitis B virus into the vaccinia core and have then infected animals with these unnatural hybrid viruses.

The scientists were delighted to discover that animals infected with the hybrids made protective antibodies against vaccinia, and also against the hepatitis virus. The same thing has been done by transplanting into vaccinia virus some key ingredients of herpes virus and flu virus.

That is the strategy some scientists are exploring against the AIDS virus.

All vaccines function by presenting to the body's internal defenses something harmless that the body will recognize as foreign and will make protective antibodies against. Although vaccinia virus is totally distinct from smallpox virus, it does carry on its surface something that the immune system recognizes both on vaccinia and on smallpox virus particles. Thus, the vaccine protects against either or both.

Experts estimate there is room in the vaccinia virus DNA for insertion of at least a dozen foreign genes. Incorporation of these foreign genes could transform the vaccinia virus into a multipurpose vaccine that might protect, for example, against herpes, hepatitis, and conceivably even some important nonvirus diseases as well. Gonorrhea and malaria are possible examples.

Some public-health experts who helped eradicate smallpox from the world are enthusiastic about this new role for the oldest vaccine. Their efforts proved that vaccinia can be given almost anywhere, cheaply, efficiently, and effectively. For many diseases that plague the Third World, it seems ideal.

But there is controversy about the possible new uses of vaccinia. One in about 100,000 people who receive the vaccine develops a serious reaction, sometimes including encephalitis.

Vaccinia virus also involves a strange problem that is partly psychological and partly political as well as medical. In various preparations the virus has been used effectively for almost 200 years against smallpox. But this experience, a success story that is almost certainly without equal in medicine, has also demonstrated clearly that rare but serious complications can occur. Sometimes they are fatal. In countries such as the United States, where strict vaccination had eliminated smallpox totally from their territories decades ago, routine vaccination of children was given up because it had actually become a greater health hazard than smallpox itself. That is to say, once smallpox had been eradicated, the disease itself was no longer a health hazard at all; yet a handful of children continued to suffer from the side effects of the live vaccinia virus in the vaccine. Some of these cases were unexplainable, but more often they were cases in which the vaccinia virus grew and caused disease of its own because the person who received the vaccine had a faulty immune defense system that could not withstand even something as relatively harmless as vaccinia virus.

In countries where smallpox had been a real threat until recently, it was sometimes difficult for public-health officials to take the unprecedented step of halting vaccination, even though they knew it was protection against a disease that no longer exists. As one expert put it, after smallpox was eradicated, another public-health campaign was needed to eradicate vaccination.

The extremely small, but real, safety problem with vaccinia virus is the main reason why some experts doubt the wisdom of redesigning the virus to fight new wars against disease. The risks were well worth taking when the alternative was something disfiguring and deadly like smallpox, these experts argue, but certainly widespread use of vaccinia would not be worth the risk against something less important — the common cold, to take an extreme example.

Those scientists who are doing the vaccinia work are confident that the remodeled virus can be made far safer than the safest strains that have been used in smallpox vaccination programs, but public health is always a balancing of risk against benefit. With vaccinia, opinions differ on how that balance stands.

The irony of the situation is that there are large regions of our planet, mostly in the Third World, where infectious and parasite diseases are still desperately important. Under such circumstances, vaccinia retooled to protect against hepatitis B virus, and perhaps polio and malaria as well, would seem to be clearly worthwhile. In poverty-stricken societies babies born with faulty immune defenses seldom survive infancy anyway, and the other kinds of one-in-a-million adverse effects of vaccinia would be eclipsed in significance by the millions of people who would be spared serious disease by virtue of vaccination.

But today, leaders of the Third World are understandably resentful of having the industrialized nations send them things that are not deemed fit for use at home. Many conscientious people in the developed countries take the same view. Will vaccinia virus fall victim to this perception of a double standard? Today, no one knows.

Another issue relates to the biology of the virus and the effects that manipulating its genes might produce.

Dr. Maurice Hilleman of Merck, Sharp & Dohme, the drug company, offers the reminder that vaccinia is, after all, a live virus. Manipulating its genes in the laboratory, he suggests, might have unexpected and dangerous effects in some vaccine recipients.

Dr. Hilleman, an outspoken scientist of many years experience, is one of the world's leading experts in vaccine research. He favors a different use of gene-splicing techniques.

The concept, again, boils down to a matter of shapes: putting something into a vaccine that will make the body's immune defenses think they are encountering a natural virus.

The techniques of gene-splicing make this possible. Scientists find the gene that represents the instruction code for making a protein of the virus surface and put that gene into bacteria or yeast. The microbes then put the gene's instructions to work, becoming living factories to produce the needed substance, which can then be harvested for use as a vaccine. The product ought to be totally harmless because it contains nothing but the surface protein and no virus nucleic acid at all. Such a product could never cause a virus infection.

Scientists at Merck, collaborating with specialists at Chiron Corporation, developed just such a vaccine against the hepatitis B virus, which ranks as one of the world's foremost public-health problems. The liver infections are so numerous — at least 200 million worldwide — that the toll can be imagined only by thinking of the entire population of the United States, every man, woman, and child, as being simultaneously ill with the disease.

A good vaccine, inexpensive enough for use in the Third World, could make a profound difference to global public health. It might be a landmark in another fashion, too. Liver cancer is almost always fatal and, in some regions, including large areas of mainland China, it is the leading cause of death from cancer. In regions where hepatitis B infections are most common, liver cancer is almost always preceded by infection with the virus. It is considered a key factor in the cause of the cancers. A vaccine against hepatitis B could turn out to be the world's first effective anticancer vaccine.

Merck had already produced a safe, effective vaccine against the hepatitis B virus. It has been available commercially for more than a year under the trade name Heptavax-B and is already widely used in the United States to protect hospital workers and others who are at high risk of infection with the virus.

But Heptavax-B itself is hardly likely ever to solve the world hepatitis problem. The source of material for this highly useful vaccine explains why.

To date no one has ever succeeded in growing the hepatitis B virus in any laboratory tissue culture. Because of that, there was no way of producing material from which to make the vaccine. The drug company scientists solved this problem by allowing natural human infections in the outside world to do the job for them. When the virus grows in an infected person, it manufactures a large excess of a natural chemical that makes up part of the surface of the virus particle. This is known as the hepatitis B surface antigen. Clumps of this substance circulate in the hepatitis-infected patient's blood as tiny particles.

The vaccine makers harvest these particles from blood donated by persons who are infected "carriers" of the hepatitis B virus. After extraction from the donor blood, the surface antigen is purified to eliminate all trace of the virus itself and everything else that might be harmful. The harvested particles become the active material of the vaccine.

But, although safe and effective, the vaccine has serious disadvantages. It takes nearly a year to make a batch, and a series of three shots costs about one hundred dollars. The price is totally out of reach for the regions of the world where it is needed most.

At this point, the extraordinary new talents of the gene-splicers may be coming to the rescue.

One general principle of gene-splicing research is that if the substance can be found, so can the gene for making it. And, if that gene can be found, it ought to be possible to reproduce it and transplant that gene into some microbe that will thereupon become a factory for making the gene's product.

In many laboratories throughout the world, large glass jugs filled with milky, amber-colored fluid sit vibrating on "shake tables" to keep their contents mixing and uniform, while microbes inside perform strange feats. The microbes — bacteria in some cases, yeasts in others — have been redesigned to carry foreign genes for whatever product the genetic engineers would like to manufacture. Each such jug is a factory making a product.

In January 1984, Dr. Hilleman's group at Merck published a report in the scientific journal *Nature* saying they had grown the hepatitis B surface antigen in cells of brewer's yeast, had harvested the particles — they looked just like the particles found in human blood plasma — and had used this material to protect chimpanzees against the dangerous liver infection.

"This is the first example of a vaccine produced from recombinant cells which was effective against a human viral infection," they said in the report in *Nature*.

The project was a collaboration between the team at Merck and a scientific group in California led by Dr. William Rutter of the University of California at San Francisco and Dr. Pablo

Valenzuela of Chiron, a biotechnology company. Dr. Valenzuela is an expert in adapting yeast cells to such production uses.

A vaccine based on this research has been developed by Merck. This product, the first genetically engineered human vaccine to be licensed in the world, was approved by the Food and Drug Administration in 1986 and went on the market, under the trade name Recombivax HB, in January 1987. Whether it will prove cheaper in the long run than the conventional vaccine remains to be seen, but its successful development was evidence that a new era in vaccine design has indeed dawned.

Hepatitis vaccines produced through similar genetic engineering techniques are being developed by several other companies here and abroad. At the same time, vaccine developers are making a major effort to adapt the conventional blood-derived vaccine to a manufacturing process so inexpensive that it would be acceptable to the Third World.

The hepatitis B virus is just one among many important causes of human disease for which such genetically engineered vaccines might be produced. These products are called "subunit vaccines" because they consist of carefully selected pieces of the virus, not of whole viruses dead or alive. The active vaccine ingredients are usually protein components of the virus particles' surface. Vaccines of this kind would be relatively easy to produce and would be safer than any conventional vaccine. There would be no virus in them at all, only the laboratory-grown surface subunits.

Vaccines of this sort useful to veterinary medicine have already been developed. Cetus Corporation in California and Norden Laboratories in Nebraska have marketed an artificially made subunit vaccine against an important diarrheal disease of pigs and calves called scours. Genentech of San Francisco, one of the most successful gene-splicing companies in the United States, has collaborated with the U.S. Department of Agriculture in a research program to develop a subunit vaccine against foot-and-mouth disease. This is one of the most important virus diseases of agricultural animals in the world.

Unfortunately, subunit vaccines sometimes fail to induce strong immunity in the individuals that receive them. Exactly why this is true is not yet known for certain, but it may be a matter of shapes. Within the tight architectural constraints of the virus surface, a protein may take a different shape fom what it would have when free and separate. Perhaps this makes a difference to the way the body's immune defense system "sees" the invader.

Another new strategy of vaccine design makes maximum use of the shapes of the molecules that are important in living things. The idea was pioneered by Dr. Richard A. Lerner of Scripps Clinic in La Jolla, California, and by Dr. Eckhard Wimmer of the State University of New York at Stony Brook. The logic is deceptively simple: if the body's immune defense system makes antibodies against invading viruses on the basis of the shapes their surfaces present, why bother with the virus itself or even with its products? Why not just mimic the key shapes?

There were many who thought the idea did not have a prayer of working. While chemically proteins are really nothing more than long chains of amino acids, the components all come together in intricate forms. Would it ever be possible to learn just which portions could be used to mimic the whole virus or microbe?

Dr. Lerner and his colleagues started a few years ago with the influenza virus.

Dr. Ian A. Wilson and Dr. Don C. Wiley of Harvard, with Dr. J. J. Skehel of Britain's National Institute for Medical Research, London, had completely analyzed the three-dimensional structure of a key protein of the flu virus surface. They were not working on vaccine design in doing this, but were trying to discover just how the viruses cause infections. The protein on which their research was focused is called a hemagglutinin. It forms spikes that stick out of the roughly spherical surface of the virus. A human exposed to the influenza virus will make antibodies against the hemagglutinin. The spikes are also important in another sense: they are the parts of the virus that enable the particles to stick to a living cell and begin the process of invasion.

Analysis of the protein structure showed what precise portions were on its surface. This offered hints as to what portion might be used to elicit antibodies. Ordinarily, the antibodies are formed against something, such as that protein, that is on the virus's surface. But the problem is more complex than that would imply. The whole protein consists of hundreds of amino acids, and it was not at all clear that any short strings of eight to a dozen or so would mimic the whole well enough to stimulate immunity.

Still, it was a possibility that could be tested. Dr. Lerner's team did so using known structural and genetic blueprints to make twenty different short chains of amino acids that corresponded, altogether, to about three quarters of the protein's total. The scientists attached each of these short chains to a large carrier protein. Then they tested each one in rabbits to see if the animals would make antibodies against any of them. To their delight, the scientists found that seventeen of the twenty antibodies raised against the test chains actually reacted with the whole virus.

"In other words," said Dr. Lerner, "a short string from almost any region of a viral protein can elicit an antibody that will recognize the entire protein."

The main requirement seemed to be that they choose a piece that would be on the outside of an intricately folded protein.

Guided by this rule, scientists have used a computer to determine which portions of a protein are likely to be on the surface and therefore would make good candidates for producing a synthetic vaccine.

There are also special tricks that make it possible to do this without the computer. Such is the sophistication of today's molecular biology that an expert can simply look at the DNA code of instructions for making a protein and offer a shrewd guess as to which parts of that protein are probably on its surface.

Dr. Lerner's team has made synthetic mimics of the viruses that cause several important human diseases, including influenza and hepatitis. Unlike all virus vaccines developed during the last 200 years, these products had nothing in them at all that had ever been a part of any virus. The new products were totally artificial, concocted from ordinary off-the-shelf chemicals, inspired by imagination and guided by sophisticated knowledge. Yet these concoctions can make the body think it has encountered a natural, disease-causing virus.

Working with scientists on the West Coast, Dr. Robert Purcell and colleagues of the National Institute of Allergy and Infectious Diseases, near Washington, D.C., have protected chimpanzees against hepatitis by using an artificial string of twenty-seven amino acids that mimics just part of a surface protein of the hepatitis virus.

While the Genentech–U.S. Department of Agriculture group was developing a vaccine against foot-and-mouth disease using the more conventional techniques of gene-splicing, Dr. Lerner's group, collaborating with British animal disease experts, was making its own off-the-shelf synthetic vaccine against the same disease. It has already been successful in experiments in protecting animals against foot-and-mouth disease.

But, so far, that success has been limited to diseases of animals. Where vaccine against human disease is concerned, there is an important drawback. The short synthetic strings of amino acids are insufficient, by themselves, to induce much immune response. That is why the group at Scripps tied them to larger proteins in the original experiments. To be effective, they all seem to need something called an adjuvant, which is simply any substance that sharply accentuates the immune response. Unfortunately, today's most powerful known adjuvants are too corrosive for use in humans. They cause sores and abcesses at the point of injection. Many experts say that one of the current needs of the field is a new and better adjuvant that can be used in vaccines for humans.

The new techniques of biology also allow vaccine designers to do things deliberately that they used to do almost blindly and to discover causes that had always been obscure.

To create any live virus vaccine, it is necessary to take a virus that is known to produce disease and grow it in the laboratory until the vaccine-makers find at least one strain that has become harmless. To some extent this is a hit-or-miss process in which the real developmental work is up to the virus itself. Dr. Edwin D. Kilbourne, of Mt. Sinai Hospital and Medical School, says the process is rather like animal husbandry. The vaccine-makers grow a virus in the laboratory under abnormal conditions of temperature or of available nutrients, knowing that mutants will arise spontaneously to profit from the conditions. These mutant strains would be at a disadvantage in growing in the human body and, therefore, might make safe and effective vaccines.

Today, however, a virus's traits can be changed deliberately by deleting small, precisely known, pieces of its DNA or RNA. In short, mutations today can be made virtually to order.

Dr. Robert Chanock, of the U.S. National Institutes of Health, notes that those rare cases of paralytic polio arising from polio vaccine seem linked much more often to polio virus of type 3 than to either of the other types that go into the vaccine. For years, the reason for this was unknown. But close study of the genetic material of the polio virus by scientists in England has now explained it. The virus of type 3 that is used in the vaccine differs from the disease-causing "wild type" virus by mutational changes in only ten of the many hundreds of nucleotides in the virus's nucleic acid. In type 1, the mutations total five times as many. The case with type 2 has not yet been checked.

But the difference in mutation numbers between types 1 and 3 explains why it is easier for type 3 to revert to the wild type. A substantially smaller number of changes are needed. An important lesson from this, Dr. Chanock says, is that the new techniques of gene-splicing offer new and superior ways of modifying viruses and other causes of disease so that they make much better and safer vaccines. Again, it is a matter of mutations made to order in the laboratory.

Among the most promising examples of this kind of genetic manipulation comes from the Center for Vaccine Development at the University of Maryland School of Medicine. Dr. Myron M. Levine and Dr. James B. Kaper and colleagues have done genetic surgery on the bacteria that cause cholera. By doing this, the team has produced something they hope will become a new, and much better, vaccine against that widespread and often deadly infection.

"Despite nearly a century of effort, a satisfactory cholera vaccine is not yet a reality," said Dr. Levine and his colleagues in a recent report.

Now they have produced something superior by discovering the precise genes of the cholera germ are the keys to its production of cholera toxin — the poison through which the bacteria do their harm. The scientists have used recombinant DNA techniques to construct a new set of genetic instructions for making the key gene, but they made it defective, with most of that gene deliberately left out. They made a specific, laboratory-designed mutation. Cholera bacteria modified in this way do not produce the dangerous toxin, but they do stimulate immunity to cholera. This work, too, is a matter of benevolent trickery. The genetically modified microbes have already protected human volunteers against cholera. They represent, in the scientists' view, "the beginning of a new generation of cholera vaccines."

Malaria is at least as big a health problem throughout the world as cholera and much more complicated from the vaccine designer's point of view. It is caused by a complicated parasite that is spread by the bite of female anopheles mosquitoes. In its life cycle, the malaria parasite takes several forms. A vaccine against one is useless against all others.

Today, the two strategies used to control the disease are control of the mosquitoes that spread it and the use of drugs to combat the parasites that invade humans. Neither mosquito control nor drug treatment of patients is more than holding its own against the disease. In fact, some experts believe public-health agencies are losing ground today in the ages-old war against malaria.

The new enthusiasm for vaccines seems to be coming at just the right time. A great deal has been learned in recent years concerning the biology of the malarial parasite and of various ways to break its life cycle. Among the pioneers in this work are two doctors at New York University, Ruth and Victor Nussensweig, who have actually made an experimental vaccine that has protected animals and human volunteers against sporozoites, the stage of the malarial parasite that enters the victim's blood when an infected mosquito bites.

A problem with sporozoite vaccine, however, is that this stage of the parasite is a difficult, fast-moving target that stays in the circulating blood only an hour or less. After that, the parasite hides in its victim's liver and changes to a new form entirely.

Moreover, in order to be of any use at all, the sporozoite vaccine must be 100 percent effective. If one single sporozoite escapes destruction and gets into the liver, it will give rise to a new generation of parasites in a form called merozoite, which will emerge from the liver, sweep through the blood again, and infect red blood cells, setting up a new and difficult stage of infection. In this phase the patient is likely to become seriously ill with the alternating chills and high fevers for which malaria is known.

Scientists are working on vaccines against this stage, too, but it presents difficult problems of its own and progress is not as far advanced as the effort against the sporozoite.

Even though there are many difficulties still to be solved, vaccines against malaria are no longer considered impossible, as they were just a few years ago.

At a scientific conference on vaccines held at the Cold Spring Harbor Laboratory, Long Island, New York, Dr. Louis H. Miller, of the U.S. National Institutes of Health, said new research has led to dramatic advances in understanding and coping with the parasite. In due course, these advances should lead to the development of effective vaccines against the disease. The scientist suggested that vaccines against the sporozoite stage might be used to protect tourists and to cope with sudden epidemics of malaria; that vaccines against the merozoite stage will be used in places where malaria is widespread and seemingly entrenched; and that a third type of vaccine for humans may be developed, which would offer no direct benefit to the person who receives it, but would protect mosquitoes against the parasite. This seemingly altruistic vaccine would help break the cycle of infection from insect to human to insect and back to human again. It might prove to be an important force in curbing the disease.

Since that scientific conference, progress has been rapid. By March 1986, one vaccine against the sporozoite stage of the malarial parasite had already reached the point of safety testing in humans. It passed that test, but was disappointing to some of the scientists involved because it produced a lower level of antibodies than had been hoped. A year later, tests in humans began with a second sporozoite vaccine. No one could say with any assurance just how soon the first safe and protective malaria vaccine would arrive on the public-health scene, but, to the experts, it now seemed clearly to be no longer a question of "whether" but simply "when." The public-health implications seem vast.

Doctors and biologists in many related fields say the horizons for vaccine research and development offer a dazzling panorama of opportunities today.

Vaccines were a new and exciting horizon in Dr. Jenner's day, too, and in Dr. Pasteur's day as well. Those two main pioneers of the field would certainly be amazed at the strategies being pursued today, but above all they would be very much pleased. For, in a sense, they started it all.

Chapter Seven

Five Disorders:
Frustration and Progress

By Daniel Kagan

Daniel Kagan is the author of Cocaine: Seduction and Solution, Mute Evidence, *and numerous magazine articles on science and health topics.*

Five medical disorders stand out starkly as illustrations of the magnitude and diversity of the health problems facing the modern world. They speak of the subtle progress, often so piecemeal and slow that it goes unnoticed, that is constantly being made against them. In a sense, though, they are also quite humbling in an age when mankind has grown almost complacent about disease and tends to assume that for every illness the medical people in the white coats have a simple shot, pill, or nostrum that will instantly cure all.

Cheap, effective vaccines and antibiotic treatments for formerly dread diseases like polio, diphtheria, and smallpox lead many of us to think that terrifying, untreatable, communicable infections are a thing of the past. However, acquired immune deficiency syndrome (AIDS) serves to recall, at least in part, how medieval men must have felt when confronted with the Black Death. Facing an unstoppable and nearly always fatal disease of unknown origin and means of transmission is a sobering lesson in the power and mystery of natural biological forces. The astonishingly rapid and impressive research gains against AIDS, however, are a heartening indication of how well we can mount an effective response against even the most baffling illness.

The disorders here involve pathology on an enormous scale. Between 1.5 million and 4 million Americans carry the AIDS virus, and 10 million more may carry it worldwide; diabetes claims 10 million victims; herpes 40 million; and stroke 3 million; the elderly number 23 million, including 2 million suffering from Alzheimer's disease. These are all victims of chronic afflictions: these disease states are permanent, incurable, and, in some cases, progressive. They are states in which the definition of health ceases to be straightforward well-being and comes to be instead a measure of how effective are the therapeutic bulwarks against further deterioration. For diabetes, stroke, herpes and the diseases of aging, the word *cure* does not apply, but the word *prevention* may, and new methods of slowing the disease processes are often greeted with as much elation as are cures for other disorders. However, treatment and cure, along with prevention, are the most important words in the battle against AIDS.

One major mystery to be unraveled by modern medicine is the arcane and bedevilingly complicated operation of the immune system. Not surprisingly, four of the illnesses here — diabetes, AIDS, herpes, and Alzheimer's disease — seem to involve some shortfall or malfunction of the immune system, or some odd quirk of virus behavior that thwarts its otherwise astonishing effectiveness. Learning about these diseases means learning more about the immune system, so advances here will mean gains to be applied elsewhere, too.

These disorders also call up the newly unbottled genie of genetic engineering. Bacteria with altered DNA produce insulin for diabetics, and gene-splicing is used to grow cultures and to make experimental vaccines for herpes and AIDS. Genetic-engineering techniques have also yielded the most promising recent advances in the understanding of Alzheimer's disease.

The diseases here also serve to remind that not all medical practice and research take place at the level of chromosomes, viruses, and cell-mediated immune reactions invisible to the naked eye. They are good illustrations of how the disease process fits into the interplay between the microworld of vaccines and hormone-receptor activity, and the macroworld of social forces and human behavior.

The transmission of AIDS, for instance, largely depends not on some supernaturally infectious tendency of its causative virus, but on learned and modifiable behaviors: promiscuous homosexual sex, intravenous drug abuse, and high-risk sex practices among heterosexuals. Changes in these social factors within the homosexual community have already apparently altered the spread of the disease there.

The most prevalent form of diabetes is also mediated largely by social factors and malleable behaviors: diet, exercise, and the handling of stress. Stroke, too, is greatly affected by these same factors, and prudent management can slow the declines of aging. Herpes can be avoided via changes in sexual and dating behavior. The individual, then, can exert some control over his susceptibility to these disorders simply by choosing the most beneficial paths of action.

Social factors also operate on the health of the elderly. Isolation, depression, and decline in meaningful involvement in work and recreational activity can damage the health of the aged. And our society's having turned the old into outcasts from the normal range of life has also turned their medical problems into a terra incognita that until recently led many doctors astray into misdiagnoses and erroneous medical treatment.

In other words, these five disorders illustrate how health and disease are outcomes of the interaction of the very large with the very small, of a minuscule virus with a sizable human, of a puny individual with a huge society, and vice versa. Other contrasts like that between the tiny and the great are to be found here: the miraculous action of the immune system against its frightening and inexplicable failures; the utter wonder of daily phenomena like insulin production and the functioning of the brain, versus beta-cell shutdown and the ravages of Alzheimer's disease and stroke; the simple gustatory pleasure of the food we eat, versus the profound effects that the molecules of its nutrients can have on diabetes, stroke, aging, and perhaps even Alzheimer's and herpes.

These five conditions show that the chronically ill person is not an isolated individual beset by disease processes, but is rather one damaged thread in a much larger tapestry, whose weave, pattern, and substance profoundly affect his state. And like a thread, his own health is made up of many tightly spun elements smaller than himself, any one of which can fail and damage his existence.

DIABETES

Of the 10 million diabetics in the United States, 90 percent suffer from type II, or adult-onset, diabetes, so called because it usually appears after age forty. This form of the disease can be managed by weight control and strict dietary regulation, and rarely requires insulin. Ten percent, or about one million people, have type I, or juvenile, diabetes, which usually strikes people below the age of twenty, comes on abruptly and with extreme symptoms, and must be controlled by daily doses of insulin.

In both cases, elevated blood glucose levels do long-term damage to blood vessels, heart, kidneys, and eyes. Diabetics are twenty-five times more prone to blindness than the average person, seventeen times more likely to develop kidney disease, forty times more likely to develop gangrene that leads to amputation, and twice as likely to have heart attacks. Diabetes causes 37,000 deaths a year in the United States. Directly and indirectly, it is reckoned that the disease takes a 5-billion-dollar yearly toll on the economy.

Both worldwide and in the United States, diabetics are proliferating faster than the rest of the population. The U.S. population increases at the rate of 1 percent annually: in recent years, the increase in American diabetics has reached 6 percent. The average American born in 1980 will have a 20 percent chance of developing the disease during his or her lifetime.

In spite of these daunting figures, and in spite of the fact that diabetes cannot be cured, only managed, the past several years have shown dramatic advances in the understanding of the disease's causes. Several promising new approaches to treatment have emerged, including a few that may lead to cures in the future.

The symptoms of diabetes (actually those of the more dramatic type I) have been described by the physicians of every society since the ancient Egyptians: great and constant thirst, excessive urination, profound and rapid weight loss despite normal appetite, eventual coma, and finally death. The symptoms of type II are subtler: rapid, unexplained weight loss, itching of the skin, drowsiness, slow healing of wounds or infections, numbness or tingling in the feet, and blurred vision. The symptoms of both types stem from abnormally elevated glucose levels in the blood. This is caused by a deficiency in the action of the hormone insulin, which triggers glucose metabolism in cells. Recent research indicates that this diminished insulin function has a different cause in each type of the disease.

The rapid onset of type I diabetes is due to a malfunction of the insulin-producing beta cells in the islets of Langerhans in the pancreas. The cells simply stop producing the insulin needed for the absorption of the heightened blood glucose levels that follow any recent meal. The body cannot convert the glucose into energy, and its buildup in the blood causes damage. Daily doses of insulin are necessary to compensate for this insulin deficiency, although diet management is also helpful.

It has recently been understood that type II diabetes is caused not by damaged beta cells and a lack of insulin, but rather by the body's inability to use the insulin released into the blood. Type II diabetics often have normal blood levels of insulin. Research at the National Institutes of Health (NIH) indicates that type II diabetics may have a shortage of insulin receptors on the surfaces of insulin-receptive cells. This makes them respond inadequately or not at all to the glucose uptake and utilization cycle that is initiated when blood-borne insulin molecules attach to the diminished number of receptor sites. The NIH work also indicates that obesity, which exists in almost all type II diabetics, decreases the number of these receptors on cells, and that dieting and weight loss can return the receptor count to normal and diminish diabetes symptoms.

There is a heredity factor, and therefore a genetic component, to type II diabetes: One-third of victims have a family history of the illness, and 85 percent of these have one diabetic parent. But it is only with recent strides in genetic research that diabetologists have begun to understand how this dimension of the disease works. One theory, advanced after study of the Pima Indians in Arizona, among whom *half* of all adults are diabetic by the age of thirty-five, posits a "thrifty gene" passed down in the Indians' line for generations. This gene would have allowed the desert-dwelling Pimas, who lived in a cycle of plenty and famine, to overload the storage capacities of their fat reserves in plentiful times, so they could survive the lean periods. In trying to piece together the Pimas' known tendency toward diabetes and overweight on a normal diet, researchers are looking for a similar genetic element in other cases of type II diabetes.

More obscure genetic, but not hereditary, factors have been found in type I diabetes as well. The key question in type I diabetes is why the number of beta cells in the pancreas suddenly diminishes to nearly zero, chocking off insulin production. Current work indicates that one reason for this may be viral infection, but since the viruses associated with type I diabetes — mumps, rubella, and Coxsackievirus B4 — commonly affect large segments of the population while only a tiny fraction end up with diabetes, researchers believe there must be a factor that predisposes these individuals toward beta-cell damage from these viruses.

Some research indicates that this special susceptibility may reside in several genes that are known to code a part of the immune system known as the histocompatibility, or HLA, system. Work in Denmark, London, New York, and Minnesota has sketched a picture of a high correlation of HLA-produced antigens — and, by association, certain genes — with type I diabetes, and a corresponding association of other HLA antigens (and therefore genes) with significant *declines* in type I diabetes. Current theory is that the first HLA gene may influence the immune system toward a deficient response to viruses that preferentially attack beta cells, while the second HLA gene might enhance the immune response to the invaders. People in whom the first HLA gene dominates would be genetically predisposed to beta-cell damage from viruses that might leave the beta cells of other people unscathed.

It has also been found that type I patients often produce antibodies to their own beta cells, which attack and destroy them as if they were foreign tissue or invading viruses or bacteria. This autoimmune reaction may also be mediated by genetic factors. The process may also be triggered by a viral infection. Canadian experiments using the immunosuppressive drug cyclosporine on type I patients showed that the drug did indeed seem to prevent this autoimmune destruction of beta cells, lending support to the theory. Though cyclosporine is too drastic a measure to be used for ongoing treatment or prevention of type I diabetes, this work may open the way for future treatments aimed at the immune system.

To date, though, incomplete understanding of the workings of the immune system and the action of genetically produced diseases has prevented the development of any treatments for either of these two seeming abnormalities. Researchers can use the HLA antigens and beta-cell autoantibodies as markers to try to identify type I diabetes sufferers. A 1983 study disclosed that the twin and triplet siblings of type I victims show the beta-cell antibodies in their blood up to three years before the disease's onset, and in 1985, a test was developed to reveal those antibodies. Such screening tests may help diagnose imminent victims and perhaps allow for early treatment to lessen the eventual impact of the disease.

New indications of the possible role of viral infections in triggering type I diabetes have been simultaneously revealing and maddeningly vague. There is a poorly understood correlation between mumps and rubella and diabetes: a tiny percentage of people who contract these illnesses will soon afterward develop type I diabetes, but the immunologic or genetic link between the two conditions is unknown. In 1978, the first real evidence of virus-induced type I diabetes was recorded when a young boy was admitted to a Washington, D.C., hospital with acute type I symptoms that followed an attack of a flulike illness. His beta cells turned out to have been destroyed by the common Coxsackievirus B4, which afflicts up to 50 percent of the population at one time or another. The reason for beta-cell sensitivity in cases like this is unknown.

While work on the causes of diabetes slowly advances, a tremendous amount of work has been done on treatments for both types. Over the short run, treatment — whether by insulin, oral antidiabetic drugs, diet management, or some combination of the three — has one goal: containing the blood glucose level within normal limits of upward and downward fluctuation, so the patient suffers neither hypoglycemia (low blood sugar) and its attendant uncomfortable and potentially dangerous symptoms, nor hyperglycemia (high blood sugar) and its risk of blood ketoacidosis, which can lead to coma and death. Day-to-day treatment thus aims to allow the diabetic to lead as normal a life as possible.

The goal of long-term treatment, however, is to prevent, delay, or diminish the damage to heart, blood vessels, eyes, nerves, and kidneys that is caused by periodically elevated blood glucose levels. This wide fluctuation is inevitable, even with traditional treatment. In recent years, though, a new approach called "tight control" has been developed. Before, type I diabetics took one large dose of insulin for the whole day, usually in the morning, and sometimes a second dose at night. But the body's glucose level and need for insulin varies sharply during the day, peaking after mealtimes. Since the one- or two-shot-per-day treatment cannot answer this variable need, the body is subject to a daily cycle of abnormally elevated glucose levels and the damage they do.

Tight control aims to keep the glucose levels within the normal range, avoiding dangerous surges in hopes that the long-term damage may be curtailed. For type I diabetics and the 20 percent of type II sufferers who must take insulin, this means careful and frequent monitoring of their blood glucose levels throughout the day and more frequent adjustments of that level with more insulin injections, up to four per day, shortly before meals.

This technique has become feasible because of the recent development of relatively inexpensive, accurate, portable, and easy-to-use home blood glucose monitoring systems. In the past, diabetics monitored their blood glucose levels by testing the glucose content of their urine, not a very accurate technique. With the new systems, the patient pricks a finger and deposits a drop of blood on a chemically treated plastic strip, which then changes color to reveal the glucose concentration. These color changes are read by eye or by machine, and the patient uses insulin injections to adjust his blood level accordingly. Such tight control is now so widespread that self-care programs to teach diabetics how to use the technique are proliferating across the country.

Recent experiments using a nasal spray rather than an injection to introduce insulin into the body may point the way to even tighter control, with less discomfort, in the future. The insulin nasal spray produces rises and falls in blood insulin levels closer to the pattern seen in normal insulin production than those that are achieved with injections. The treatment will remain experimental until researchers can answer a number of questions about its cost, its potential long-term side effects, and whether a cold or hay fever would affect it.

In late 1986, the Yale University School of Medicine and twenty-six other medical centers in the United States and Canada began recruiting insulin-dependent diabetics for an ambitious seven-year-long study to determine exactly how well tight control helps prevent the physical damage wrought by diabetes. The study involves 1,400 diabetics and will cost $153 million by the time it is completed in 1994.

Meanwhile, new techniques are being developed to heal or prevent damage from the disease. A new laser treatment, for instance, can cut by half the vision loss that afflicts hundreds of thousands of diabetics. Diabetic blindness occurs because of a condition called retinopathy, in which blood vessels that nourish the retina break down. They may leak blood or fluid, develop fragile new branches, become enlarged, or trigger the formation of scar tissue, all of which can diminish or eliminate vision. The laser treatment uses a light beam to seal leaking vessels by burning pinpoint spots on the retina. It can halt vision loss, and in some cases even improve sight. And an experimental drug called aminoguanidine has been shown in laboratory tests to protect diabetic animals against abnormal, degenerative changes in their blood vessels. The high glucose levels in the blood of diabetics cause the permanent cross-linking of proteins in blood vessels. This clogs the vessels and weakens their walls, and leads to diminished circulation and degraded kidney function. Aminoguanidine prevents this cross-linking.

The ultimate form of tight control would be a perfect reconstruction of the body's own pancreatic regulating process, in other words an artificial pancreas. The last five years have seen enormous strides toward this. In fact, there are two types of "artificial pancreas" in use. Both have drawbacks but both have shown remarkable results.

Work in an artificial pancreas has taken three distinct routes: biomechanical, biochemical, and a hybrid of the two. The biochemical approach involves the implantation of functioning beta cells into the diabetic's body, where they can continue to produce insulin. The biomechanical method involves sophisticated, miniaturized insulin pumps, which are loaded with insulin and dispense it into the blood in properly calibrated doses over a long period of time. The hybrid methods involve encasing beta cells in a semipermeable membrane and implanting them in the body. The membrane allows insulin out while preventing cell-destroying antibodies from attacking the beta cells.

Animal experiments have shown that straightforward implantation of beta cells does work for up to 100 days if the cells are specially treated beforehand to decrease the likelihood of their rejection. Other animal work has involved implanting fetal beta cells from aborted animals stopped in their development at a point where the cells begin producing insulin. For obvious ethical reasons, the second method cannot be tried with humans. Two other methods hold imminent promise, though.

One technique involves extracting only the insulin-producing cells from pancreases donated by deceased individuals, treating them to decrease chances of rejection, and implanting them. Clinical trials of this method were done in 1985 with twenty-seven diabetics. In most cases, the transplanted cells produced insulin temporarily, and one woman's transplant continued to produce a large portion of her insulin supply for more than sixteen months.

This approach has become more feasible as scientists have developed new methods of "fooling" the body's immune system into accepting transplanted foreign tissue. The other technique involves the traditional transplant of a whole pancreas from a donor, and entails the usual range of problems surrounding the rejection of a new organ. Ninety of these have been done in the past twenty years. As of 1982, nineteen of the patients were still living and nine had survived for more than a year.

The hybrid methods have involved both growing insulin-producing beta cells on the outside of a tubular piece of semipermeable membrane and then implanting it as a shunt between an artery and a vein, and encasing the cells in a semipermeable capsule and implanting it in a blood vessel. Both techniques have proved successful in animals, but only for weeks at a time. They do look good for the future, however.

The biomechanical methods — insulin pumps — have been the most successful. They are used by about 10,000 Americans, primarily type I patients who have no choice about taking insulin, but they have been tried in a few cases of serious type II diabetes that have not responded to diet. The electronic, battery-operated pumps are worn outside the body and supply a steady trickle of insulin through a needle inserted under the skin. Some of them allow the patient to press a button to deliver the necessary premeal insulin surge required to deal with the postprandial glucose rise. Despite problems with clogged tubes and the need continuously to rotate the insertion point of the needle, the pumps do well in clinical trials and actual use. Other types of pump are implanted under the skin in the abdomen or near the collarbone and lack the capacity to deliver the premeal insulin boost.

Recently, a spectacularly improved version of these implantable pumps was successfully placed into a patient at Johns Hopkins Hospital in Baltimore. Unlike earlier implantable pumps, this device has a long life — five to ten years — and is programmable. The diabetic can signal the pump to vary the amount of insulin he receives simply by holding a small radio transmitter above the skin on the abdomen under which the pump has been implanted. The patient then dials a number corresponding to a computer program, and the pump responds. The device must be refilled with insulin every three months by an external needle. The pump is a computerized titanium disk developed using technology from the National Aeronautics and Space Administration. Its design is similar to equipment used on the Mars Viking spacecraft to deliver a culture medium onto the soil of Mars.

The next advance in pumps will come when an implantable insulin sensor the size of a nickel can be combined with a still-to-be-developed membrane to protect it from being covered by scar tissue. The sensor will be able to gauge blood glucose levels and automatically adjust the pump's output.

One of the most dramatic breakthroughs has been the use of genetic engineering to produce large quantities of human insulin. In 1982, the Federal Food and Drug Administration (FDA) approved the marketing of the new product, called Humulin and produced by Eli Lilly and Company with a technique developed by Genentech, Inc. Human insulin-producing genes are spliced into the DNA of common *E. coli* bacteria, which then manufacture the hormone. Humulin was the first genetically engineered product to come into common use.

A Danish firm called NOVO has taken a different route toward making an artificial insulin, by chemically altering pork insulin so that its molecular structure exactly matches that of the human hormone.

Future drug treatments for diabetes may involve substances that can alter or manage insulin activity at the cellular level. The first step toward these drugs was the complete analysis in early 1985 of the protein precursor that human cells use to make their insulin receptors, by a team of scientists at Genentech, Inc., in California, the Memorial Sloan-Kettering Cancer Center in New York, and the University of California–Veterans Administration Medical Center in San Francisco. The analysis revealed exactly how the protein, which is made up of 1,370 amino acids, is cut in two and then joined to a duplicate pair of subunits to form an active receptor. This advance makes it possible to study the receptor functions in normal cells, and to compare them to receptor functioning in the cells of diabetics. This may reveal basic facts about the chemical nature of the disease. The advance also opens the way toward making experimental changes in insulin receptors, and correlating those changes with their chemical effects on cells. From this work, it may be possible to develop new drugs to treat diabetes.

Despite all these dramatic advances, one of the most important breakthroughs in diabetes treatment concerns one of the most basic means of managing the disease: diet. It was long accepted that simple carbohydrates, sugars like glucose, fructose, and sucrose, all had the same effect on metabolism: immediate absorption followed by a rapid rise in blood glucose. This meant that diabetics were told to avoid these foods totally. Complex carbohydrates, like those in bread, beans, rice, and potatoes, were supposed to take longer to be absorbed and to yield a slower, more moderate rise in blood glucose, something diabetics strive for in diet.

Recent findings indicate that all this is incorrect. Some simple carbohydrates, like ice cream, do nothing to blood glucose levels, while some complex carbohydrates, like white potatoes or whole-wheat bread, send the levels skyrocketing. Consequently, the rigid rules of diabetic diets have had to be modified, and it is now understood that *which* complex carbohydrates patients eat is critical. Diabetics also can now eat some of the forbidden simple carbohydrates they used to shun. These findings also reveal that different combinations of complex carbohydrates act in unpredictable ways and must be carefully matched.

The new diet findings have also resulted in the replacement of the old high animal-protein, high fat, low carbohydrate diabetic regimen with a high complex-carbohydrate, high fiber diet. This approach has been recommended by the American Diabetes Association. The new diet has helped some insulin-using type II patients reduce their dependence on insulin, because it moderates glucose level swings. Some patients have used the diet to eliminate insulin completely. In addition, the lower animal-fat content reduces the odds of cholesterol-clogged arteries, a problem more prevalent among diabetics than the general population, and the high fiber intake appears to increase the number of cellular insulin receptors, thus working directly on one of the causes of type II diabetes.

There is, however, another side to all this. Because type II diabetes is so much less acute than type I, it is often very difficult to diagnose, indeed even to notice. Consequently, there are probably millions of Americans who are unaware they have the disease and who are not treating it, while it slowly wreaks havoc on their bodies. Added to this are the recent discoveries that lack of exercise and stress-related hormones can amplify the condition in people prone to diabetes. This means that the advances made in understanding and managing the disease may be undercut by the hidden, creeping increase in the number of unknowing victims. Diabetes groups have initiated intensive public awareness programs in recent years to alert people to the disease's symptoms and motivate them to seek diagnoses and treatment.

AIDS

The story of acquired immune deficiency syndrome (AIDS), first recognized in 1981, is extremely short in the time span of medical history. It is a frenzied story as well, and has become one of medical science's greatest mysteries.

The identification in the spring of 1984 of its infectious agent, a virus, or more specifically, a retrovirus known initially as HTLV-III or LAV, and the subsequent development of a cheap, reliable screening test to identify quickly the victims of the disorder, marked the end of only the first chapter. Several more critical phases must still be completed. They include the development of a vaccine and, most important, the discovery of an effective treatment. Although one drug, azidothymidine, or AZT, was approved by the FDA for limited use against AIDS, it is not a cure. It merely seems to prolong the lives and partially restore the general health of some AIDS victims. AZT does not kill the AIDS virus throughout the body, and its side effects can be devastating.

So while work continues on a number of other possible treatments, AIDS remains irreversible. And though it is possible to treat the individual infections and cancers to which its victims become vulnerable, the underlying immune deficiency is incurable. This means that right now the fate of most AIDS patients is a string of infections over a period of about two years, until they finally succumb to one of them. The mortality rate among newly diagnosed patients is 40 percent. Among cases diagnosed two or more years ago, it is virtually 100 percent.

The battle against AIDS has been as much an exercise in public health as it has been one in clinical medical research. There has been at least as much detective work as cell-culturing. And though the most dramatic breakthroughs, like the identification of the causative virus, have been the result of laboratory sleuthing, they continue to be preceded by and supported by a huge public-health investigation effort that by now spans scores of countries across the globe.

Similarly, the roadblocks to overcoming AIDS exist not only in the microworld of cell study and immune system activity, but also in the larger worlds of public perception and private behavior. Although it initially appeared that AIDS might be confined within the narrow circle of high-risk groups in which it first appeared — sexually promiscuous male homosexuals, bisexual men, needle-using drug abusers, hemophiliacs, a tiny fraction of blood transfusion recipients, the children of mothers with AIDS or who fall into any of the risk groups, and the sex partners of members of risk groups — it is now clear that AIDS is spreading into the general population.

At first, it was thought that AIDS was transmitted only through intimate sexual contact involving the contamination of one partner's blood by the other's semen, or by the direct contamination of the victim's blood by AIDS-laden blood or blood products, as when drug users share syringes, or when an AIDS-infected woman is pregnant and passes the disease to her unborn child. It is easy to see that the two largest risk groups — homosexual men, who account for about 71 percent of AIDS victims, and IV drug users, who account for about 17 percent — put themselves at risk through their sexual and drug-using behavior. It was originally thought that a change in these behaviors would substantially reduce the number of AIDS victims by severing two of the main routes of the disease's transmission: contaminated needles shared by IV drug users, and homosexual anal intercourse, which causes tears in rectal tissues, opening the way for AIDS-infected semen to enter the blood.

But findings over the past two years, along with research in

Africa, have confirmed that AIDS is also spread by normal heterosexual intercourse. This means that AIDS picked up by the sex partners of high-risk carriers can then be spread to anyone they subsequently have sex with. It seems that the primary crossover population from high-risk AIDS victims to the general public is the partners of IV drug users, and to a lesser degree the wives and female lovers of bisexual men. Since anyone can be infected with the virus for five years or longer before symptoms appear — if they ever do — subsequent sex partners of these people, and their subsequent sex partners, ad infinitum, can be infected with AIDS and spread it far and wide before realizing they have the disease. To date, no one is sure how easily AIDS is transmitted via heterosexual contact. But it is certain that the only way to avoid heterosexual spread is with the same methods of "safe sex" — the use of condoms during all sex acts in order to avoid the exchange of bodily fluids, and the total avoidance of practices like anal intercourse — recommended to those in high-risk groups.

Despite an intense surge of interest and fear about a general spread of AIDS, no one knows how many heterosexuals have already been exposed to the virus, nor does anyone know how many people will adopt routine "safe sex" as a way to protect themselves.

AIDS occurs worldwide, with a rising incidence in Canada and Western Europe, and in a long-established belt stretching across Central Africa through Uganda and Zaire. It is now generally agreed that the AIDS virus originated in Africa, where it may have mutated into its current virulent form, possibly from a similar monkey virus that spread to humans, or was introduced from the countryside, where it was unnoticed and spread slowly, into the city because of migrations over the past decade. It is thought that in the cities of Africa, carriers and victims were concentrated and the virus spread through prostitution and heterosexual contact. Then one or several things happened. The virus was brought to Belgium and France by Europeans who had Zairian or Ugandan sex partners, and from there was introduced into the American gay population. Possibly, it was carried from France to Haiti, where it established itself and was then spread to the American gay community by Haitian male prostitutes who gave it to vacationing American gays. It is also possible that the disease was picked up by Cuban soldiers stationed in Africa and carried back to the Caribbean, where it eventually made its way to Haiti and the United States.

AIDS first caught the attention of the American medical community in the summer of 1981. Since the disorder is characterized by a near-total suppression of certain functions of the immune system, it has no outward symptoms of its own. Rather, it opens its victims to infection by certain cancers that are usually very rare, and to "opportunistic" infections by a menagerie of bacteria, protozoans, fungi, viruses, and parasites that normally will not affect people with healthy immune systems.

Physicians at the federal Centers for Disease Control (CDC) in Atlanta noticed that since 1979 there had been an abnormally high incidence of a rare skin cancer called Kaposi's sarcoma, and of a parasitic and hard-to-treat lung infection called *Pneumocystitis carinii,* among highly promiscuous homosexual men. Almost immediately, they realized they faced an entirely new medical problem. Kaposi's sarcoma was nearly unheard of in men under fifty, and the classic progression of the disease involves slow development, good response to chemotherapy, and a survival rate of five to ten years. The young gay Kaposi's sarcoma patients had a rapidly advancing form of the cancer that often involved internal organs and was usually fatal. The rare pneumonia was almost never encountered in people with healthy immune systems. In fact, both diseases are common among people with suppressed immune systems: cancer patients debilitated by chemotherapy and organ transplant patients taking immunosuppressant drugs.

Researchers quickly determined that AIDS involved a drastic reduction in the number of cells called T-lymphocytes, white blood cells that fight off the cells of infectious agents or help destroy cancer cells before they multiply. The remaining T-cells are deformed. AIDS also entails an almost total lack of T-helper cells, which are produced by T-cells and further activate other components of the immune system. Finally, the number of T-suppressor cells, which inhibit the T-cell/T-helper cell production and control the extent of the immune response, remain at their normal levels. This means that an AIDS patient's immune system has the tendency not to react effectively to infections, and also to turn itself off before it starts. The normal ratio is two T-helpers to one T-suppressor cell. In AIDS this relationship is reversed.

Initially, 94 percent of the victims were highly promiscuous gay men, some of whom reported 1,000 or more sex partners per year, in contrast to the average homosexually active men who reported 500 or less, and who seemed less susceptible to AIDS. Intense research into the possible factors at work revealed that the trauma of repeated anal sex, which often results in sores or bleeding, provided an avenue for the blood of these men to become contaminated by the blood or semen of their partners. A blood-borne infectious agent would be transmitted this way, as would one carried in the semen. In addition, animal experiments have shown that semen or sperm entering the blood causes both a marked formation of antibodies and a strong overall suppression of the immune response. The added possibility that oral sex would allow the agent to enter through sores in the mouth led researchers to conclude, even this early, that AIDS might be caused by a virus that could be transmitted. Initial attention focused on two members of the herpes virus family, cytomegalovirus and Epstein-Barr virus, since almost all homosexual men show antibody evidence of having been infected by them.

By the summer of 1982, the original forty-one cases of AIDS had ballooned to 335 cases. One hundred thirty-six of the victims were dead. More people had already died from AIDS than from the highly publicized epidemics of legionnaire's disease and toxic shock syndrome. Intravenous drug users had been identified as the second largest risk group, adding support to the idea of a blood-borne agent. This was further bolstered by the appearance of AIDS in a handful of hemophiliacs, who must regularly take injections of Factor VIII, a blood-clotting substance manufactured from the extracts of thousands of blood donors, some of whom might be AIDS carriers. An inordinately high incidence of AIDS showed up among Haitian immigrants, mostly men, who almost universally denied being homosexual or using intravenous drugs. AIDS appeared among heterosexual women who were the sexual partners of high-risk men: bisexuals exposed to AIDS in the gay community or intravenous drug users. This indicated AIDS is spread by heterosexual contact and could also be caught from people with no visible symptoms of the disorder, like many of these women's sex partners.

CDC epidemiologists were also able to trace a cluster of nineteen AIDS cases and discover that nine of the victims had had sexual contact with other victims, as well as with AIDS victims in other cities. This "L.A. cluster" was one more indication that the disease was caused by a transmissible agent. And in December 1982 Dr. James Oleske, a pediatrician at St. Michael's Medical Center in Newark, New Jersey, reported that eight newborn infants and young children thirty months old or less who had developed AIDS may have caught the disease by "casual contact" with high-AIDS-risk family members — homosexuals or IV drug abusers — touching, kissing, and eating from common utensils. This contributed to a growing fear that AIDS might be spreading into the general population via routes other than blood mixing or sexual contact. Oleske's conclusions were later faulted when it was found that several of the mothers of the AIDS-afflicted children were either IV drug users or had sexual relationships with high-AIDS-risk individuals, making it likely the mothers had contracted AIDS or were carrying it and had passed it to their children while they were in the womb. The delayed onset in some of the children followed AIDS's long incubation period, which can be five years or longer.

At that point 800 cases had been reported, of which 300 (38 percent) had died. Increased media coverage and the growing fear that the disease would spread to the general public spurred Congress and the NIH to begin allotting substantial funding for AIDS research.

Meanwhile, researchers had narrowed their focus to a new retrovirus discovered in 1980 by Dr. Robert Gallo at the National Cancer Institute. Called human T-cell leukemia virus or HTLV, it was the first virus conclusively shown to cause cancer — a form of leukemia. Because the virus was so exclusively attracted to T-cells, because it is also known to cause immunosuppression, and because there is a high incidence of HTLV leukemia in the West

Indies, where Haiti is located, Gallo's team went after HTLV as the infectious agent in AIDS.

At the same time, other researchers were trying to treat AIDS with interferon and interleukin-2, antiviral substances produced by the body, while still others tried bone marrow transplants. All had minimal or transitory effects on AIDS-related infections, but none of them reversed the profound suppression of the immune system.

By May 1983, 1,450 cases of AIDS had been logged, and 558 of the victims were dead. A "doubling phenomenon" was noted: the number of AIDS cases doubled every six months. No one knew where it would stop, but even modest projections forecast tens of thousands of victims within two years. A panic was building that AIDS had contaminated the national blood supply and people stopped giving blood under the mistaken notion they could somehow contract AIDS that way. The Red Cross officially asked high-risk individuals not to donate blood. The U.S. Public Health Service declared AIDS to be its "number one priority" and earmarked $14.5 million for AIDS research in 1983, over the $7 million already committed. Inside the homosexual community, leaders worked to convince gay men to curtail excessive sexual activity to avoid contracting AIDS.

The mystery of the high AIDS incidence among Haitians began to crumble when it was revealed that one-third of Haitian men in Haiti with the disease admitted to working as homosexual prostitutes servicing American gays on vacation there, yet did not see themselves as homosexual. They were merely poor, needed money for their families, and did it for cash. The possibility now arose that many of the Haitian AIDS victims in the United States might have contracted the disease in a similar way, or from a woman who had been a sex partner of a man who acted as a homosexual prostitute.

Researchers quickly found antibodies to HTLV in the blood of some AIDS victims, and DNA from the virus in the blood of others. Gallo's team had found that the HTLV associated with AIDS was different from the virus that causes T-cell leukemia (HTLV-I and HTLV-II) and named it HTLV-III. At the same time a research team at the Pasteur Institute in Paris had isolated from

AIDS victims a similar T-cell-tropic retrovirus that they called lymphadenopathy virus or LAV. LAV got its name from the condition of lymphadenopathy, a swelling of the lymph nodes seen as an early stage of AIDS and often called pre-AIDS.

In July 1983 national blood reserves had dropped to a perilously low level because of the continuing fear that blood donations could transmit AIDS. A federal AIDS information hotline opened and received 5,000 calls a day. The blood shortage was turned around only when it was made clear that AIDS caught from contaminated blood accounted for only about ten cases out of the 10 million transfusions performed over the past three years. Still, hospital workers feared handling AIDS patients and sometimes neglected them, some police officers refused to handle physically suspects with AIDS without donning masks and gloves, and in New York undertakers refused to embalm AIDS victims until they got strict guidelines from the state health department. Even some physicians and medical students worried about contracting the disease and refused to treat AIDS patients.

By August 1983, former Health and Human Services Secretary Margaret Heckler asked Congress to raise the funding for AIDS research to $40 million. The number of cases stood at 1,972, and 759 of those victims were dead.

By now, AIDS had been reported in thirty-three countries, and most researchers concurred that it was probably many times more prevalent than it was visible, with hundreds of thousands of victims worldwide and tens of thousands in the United States who were either in the incubation period or had caught the disease and did not succumb to it or develop full-blown cases. The doubling phenomenon began to level off. By the end of 1983, 3,000 cases had been reported, 1,283 of those were dead and the mortality rate for cases diagnosed two years before was approximately 100 percent.

In January 1984, researchers at the University of California isolated a previously unknown retrovirus from monkeys with a disease similar to AIDS, called simian AIDS or SAIDS. The virus was so similar to HTLV that the discovery suggested the human agent might be isolated the same way. The researchers used the

SAIDS virus to infect healthy monkeys, proving it was blood-borne and indicating its human counterpart might also be.

In April 1984, the French research team at the Pasteur Institute under Dr. Luc Montagnier reported it had found its LAV virus in 80 to 90 percent of the blood samples from American AIDS victims that the CDC had sent them for analysis. It appeared the causative agent had finally been isolated, but time and more tests were needed to confirm this. At the same time, the American team under Dr. Gallo announced that it had determined its target virus, HTLV-III, to be the cause of AIDS. They had isolated it from one-third of the blood samples of AIDS patients and from 90 percent of the samples from a pool of patients with pre-AIDS. Gallo's team had also perfected a way to culture AIDS-infected T-cells so they could be studied and used for further tests.

Gallo's team had also isolated antibodies to HTLV-III from 88 percent of the blood samples of their AIDS subjects and 79 percent of the samples of the pre-AIDS subjects.

Most researchers quickly understood that LAV and HTLV-III were probably the same retrovirus or, at most, different strains of the same virus. Work could now begin on a test to diagnose AIDS victims early in the disease and to screen blood donors from contaminating the blood supply. The cell-culture technique meant that work could begin on a vaccine. Estimates of two to five years for the vaccine and six months for the screening test were put forth. The federal government had spent $75 million on AIDS research since 1981, with an additional $54 million set for 1985 alone. The number of cases stood at 4,087, of which 1,758 had died.

By September 1984, the Chiron Corporation in California had successfully cloned the genetic material from both the HTLV-III and LAV retroviruses. The next step would be to splice this material into the DNA of bacteria to create microbial factories to produce AIDS virus substances to be used to develop the vaccine and screening test. In early October, researchers isolated HTLV-III from the semen and saliva of AIDS victims, but there is no proof that saliva is a means of transmission for the disease.

Finally, in late October, researchers were able to infect

chimpanzees with human AIDS by injecting them with the virus, a step vital for vaccine research. An NIH team used HTLV-III to do this, and a CDC team used the LAV. As with human viral infections, only a percentage of the infected animals came down with AIDS: the others appeared to fight it off. The CDC noted that research so far indicated that up to 250,000 people in the United States, past and present, may have been similarly infected with HTLV-III but that only a small percentage had, or would ever, develop the disease. It was projected that up to 10 percent of this population might develop AIDS, a total of about 25,000.

From this point to the present, research on treatments and a vaccine for AIDS, attempts to limit its spread, and our overall understanding of the virus have all accelerated at a breakneck rate. The news that AIDS is spreading into the heterosexual population, the release of official estimates that 1.5 million Americans may be infected with AIDS, and the prediction that the United States may have 270,000 cases of active AIDS by 1991, which by then may cause 54,000 deaths annually, have all caused AIDS to displace heart disease as the number two health worry for Americans, after cancer. Several candidates from both major parties have declared that funding for AIDS research, and policies to halt its spread, will be major issues in the 1988 presidential election.

This intense concern is not limited to the United States. AIDS has been reported in ninety-one countries and it is believed to infect up to 10 percent of the population of some African nations. The World Health Organization (WHO) has suggested that up to 10 *million* people around the world may carry the AIDS virus.

All this, along with the disease's incurability and its 100 percent mortality rate among those who begin to exhibit its symptoms, makes AIDS perhaps the most dangerous infectious health hazard in the world today. It may also be the greatest challenge ever encountered by modern medical research.

There have been scores of significant developments and setbacks in the battle against AIDS over the past three years. They can best be tracked as a running chronology under three headings:

¶What has been learned about its spread, and the efforts being made or considered for curtailing it;

¶Research toward developing treatments and cures;
¶Research toward developing vaccines.

Spread

In October 1984, the city of San Francisco moved to limit the spread of AIDS by closing all its bathhouses catering to male homosexuals. This was done to stop the high-risk sexual activity taking place in the bathhouses. In November 1984, the bathhouses were reopened, but with strict, court-ordered limitations on the types of sexual behavior that could take place in them, to be enforced by monitoring employees hired specially for that purpose. This set a precedent for similar actions to halt the spread of AIDS that were later taken in New York City.

By April 1985, a test to screen donated blood for the presence of antibodies to the AIDS virus had been developed and put into use. Now a means was finally at hand to keep new AIDS-contaminated blood from entering the nation's blood supply and to prevent further spread of AIDS through contaminated blood given in transfusions. Even at this early stage, many people expressed concern that a positive test result could stigmatize the individual if it became known — even though the presence of antibodies means only that the person has been exposed to the HTLV-III virus, and does not mean he has active AIDS or will ever get it — and emphasized the critical importance of maintaining the confidentiality of such test results. The test yields a fairly high rate of false positives (up to 1 percent). This serves as a kind of built-in safety buffer, but also presents some problems. Soon afterward, a second, more expensive, and time-consuming test called the Western blot was developed. The practice became to back up any positives with a more accurate Western blot test, and to classify as true positives only those who register antibodies on the backup test, too.

Concern over the disease's spread heightened soon afterward when a CDC study revealed that the HTLV-III virus could persist in infected people for at least five years without giving rise to any symptoms, yet could be spread by such symptomless carriers as easily as it could be spread by those with symptoms. This meant that people who did not know they were infected could pass AIDS to others, who would have no outward way of knowing that their sex partner placed them at risk. The finding underlined the critical need for all high-risk people to take the AIDS antibody blood test.

By the summer of 1985, The CDC had recorded 11,271 AIDS cases altogether, of whom 5,641 had died. It became obvious at that time that the number of infants and young children with AIDS was rising. More and more women, infected with the virus through their own IV drug use or through sex with male partners in high-risk groups, were passing AIDS to their unborn babies in the womb or infecting them during birth. By July, there were 600 children nationwide who had AIDS or a constellation of pre-AIDS symptoms called AIDS-related complex or ARC. Many of these mothers did not know they had been infected with the disease until their children showed symptoms. These child AIDS victims also revealed that the heterosexually spread AIDS afflicting their mothers was becoming disproportionally centered among the poorer black and Hispanic communities, which have a higher concentration of IV drug users than society at large. AIDS children also began appearing in more middle-income groups, thus revealing that their mothers had been heterosexually infected by bisexual mates or those who had kept IV drug use secret.

By August, the NIH reported that through the use of the new AIDS screening test, the nation's blood supply was now virtually free of AIDS-contaminated blood. The only lingering concern, experts said, was that those who had had transfusions before testing began might have received infected blood, and would not know it for several years because of the disease's potentially long dormancy period.

Meanwhile, the increase of AIDS outside the risk groups had sparked a wave of fear among heterosexuals. Experts, including those at the CDC, repeatedly stressed that only 1 percent of the 12,599 AIDS cases recorded to date were caused by heterosexual transmission, and that almost all those victims were women who had contracted it from bisexual men or IV drug users. They emphasized that AIDS did not appear to be jumping into the general population, and that the risk of infection from one contact with a high-risk individual, like a drug-using prostitute, was low.

The strongest assurances came from studies indicating that it is virtually impossible to contract AIDS through casual contact, such as sharing toothbrushes or eating utensils, or drinking from the same cup. However, one more danger in the heterosexual transmission of AIDS was recognized when a medical team in Australia reported that four women there had apparently been infected with the virus through artificial insemination with sperm from an infected donor.

The Pentagon announced that it would begin screening millions of prospective military recruits for exposure to AIDS, and later expanded this testing to all 2.1 million U.S. military personnel. Though assurances were made that test results would be kept confidential, the mandatory testing of such a large group of people, along with the increasing numbers of people voluntarily taking the test, brought into focus the issue of the right to confidentiality of test results, versus society's need to identify carriers of a fatal disease and possibly to track their partners.

In similar instances in the past, public-health requirements have superseded individual rights. Other sexually transmitted diseases like gonorrhea and syphilis are required to be reported and are routinely tracked. Accessible records are kept of victims of transmissible illnesses like tuberculosis. But none of these diseases is 100 percent fatal or carries the stigma of AIDS, so none of them has engendered such an intense desire for total confidentiality by those found to be infected. This concern became even greater since a number of major insurance companies made it clear that they would like to screen AIDS carriers, and even uninfected people in high-risk groups, in order to deny them health and life insurance. This issue is still being hashed out, amid proposals for widespread mandatory testing and recommendations for harsh new laws to ensure confidentiality by requiring imprisonment and heavy fines for anyone who breaches the confidentiality of AIDS test subjects.

By October, it became clear that the demographics of the spread of AIDS had begun to shift, at least in areas like New York, which hold the highest concentrations of AIDS victims. The percentage of new reported AIDS cases among homosexual men in New York had dropped from 76 percent of the total in 1981 to only 58 percent in 1985, because of organized efforts in the gay community to stop the epidemic. At the same time, the percentage of new cases among IV drug users in New York had almost doubled, from 18 percent in 1981 to 33 percent in 1985. Little hope was expressed that the unorganized drug-abuser community, which is also predominantly poor, black, and Hispanic, could mount successful anti-AIDS tactics. But a number of programs were begun in New York and New Jersey to try to educate addicts not to share needles, to clean their needles with laundry bleach and water before using them, and to use condoms to avoid spreading or contracting AIDS.

And to combat the spread of AIDS in the heterosexual community, many colleges and universities instituted programs to educate students about safe sexual practices.

By November, WHO reported AIDS in seventy-one countries, up from forty countries in August. Central Africa — particularly Zaire, Uganda, Rwanda, Burundi, and Zambia — had become the focus of attention because research revealed that AIDS was spreading throughout the general population there primarily via heterosexual intercourse, and was affecting as many women as men. African medical practices, such as not sterilizing needles between uses, and the fact that the African blood supply appeared to be highly contaminated with AIDS also seemed to be contributing factors.

Yet very few AIDS cases had been officially reported in Africa, in part because many African governments denied the disease was a problem there and resented the theory that AIDS had begun in Africa. But AIDS had been so widespread there for so long that it was even called by the slang name "Slim" in parts of Uganda, where it is common. Blood tests done on old, stored blood samples had recently revealed that the AIDS virus, or one similar to it, was present in Africa in the 1970s, and possibly as early as the 1960s.

In December, after persistent pressure, several major African countries finally began to acknowledge the AIDS problem there, and to report cases and support a new effort begun by WHO to help developing countries build health systems designed to detect AIDS.

In the first few months of 1986, the federal government stepped up its efforts to curtail the spread of AIDS. The Department of Health and Human Services proposed regulations requiring all potential immigrants to the United States to take the AIDS blood test, and barring all those who tested positive. President Reagan ordered Surgeon General Dr. C. Everett Koop to prepare a major report on the disease. The following month, the AIDS coordinator for the U.S. Public Health Service recommended that the millions of Americans in high-risk groups all undergo periodic AIDS blood tests. By then, the CDC had recorded 18,070 cases of AIDS, of which at least 9,691 had died. A study in California revealed around this time that the data on the distribution of AIDS might be inadequate, because physicians there were under-reporting, by from 17 percent to 35 percent, the number of their patients who had died from AIDS. This was being done, the physicians said, to avoid the stigma associated with the disease, and to sidestep the refusal of some insurance companies to honor the claims of victims and the reluctance of some funeral homes to embalm victims.

By June, the CDC had recorded 21,517 cases of AIDS and 11,713 deaths from the disease. Then the U.S. Public Health Service released a set of projections based on existing data that dwarfed those figures, and shocked the country. The service estimated that 1 million to 1.5 million Americans had already been infected by the AIDS virus and were potential carriers. By 1991, 20 to 30 percent of them would develop the disease, while AIDS would spread widely outside risk groups and concentrated AIDS pockets like New York and San Francisco.

In 1991, the agency predicted, 74,000 new cases of AIDS would be diagnosed, there would be a cumulative total of 270,000 cases of active AIDS, and 179,000 deaths from all cases known to date. One to 2 percent of these would be heterosexuals, while the existing distribution of victims — about 70 percent homosexual and bisexual men and about 25 percent IV drug users — would continue. Up to 54,000 people would die from AIDS in 1991 alone, more than were killed in the Vietnam war, and patient care would cost between $8 billion and $16 billion per year. The primary route of transmission into the heterosexual community, the agency said, would be through IV drug users and their sexual partners.

In the face of these projections, federal and state health officials recommended a broad, aggressive national effort to educate people about avoiding AIDS risks, and to prepare the nation for the onslaught of new AIDS patients.

A few weeks later, a team studying the spread of AIDS in Haiti reported that the predominant route of transmission there was now heterosexual contact. In 1983, 71 percent of victims there were members of the known high-risk groups. Now, however, only 11 percent were, while 72 percent of AIDS cases were among heterosexuals who said they did not fall into any known high-risk category, as opposed to 22 percent in 1983. The shift may have been an indication of what could happen in the United States over the next several years.

By October, WHO reported a sharp increase in reported AIDS cases worldwide, to 31,646, from 20,476 at the beginning of the year. It was estimated that there might be as many as 50,000 cases, as yet unreported, in Africa. A month later, WHO announced it was beginning a coordinated, global effort to combat AIDS, which it characterized as "a health disaster of pandemic proportions." WHO spokesmen said that, worldwide, 100,000 people have come down with AIDS, 1 million have AIDS-related disorders, and up to 10 million are infected with the virus and are presumably capable of spreading the disease. They also said that as many as 100 million people could be infected within five years.

Surgeon General C. Everett Koop finally delivered his report on AIDS, and rocked many of his conservative supporters by declaring that a huge national effort at AIDS education should be undertaken, and that it should include frank instruction to elementary school children about unsafe sex practices and the role of drug abuse in spreading AIDS. Dr. Koop, a staunch foe of abortion and no supporter of birth control, also came out for condom ads on television to promote the value of condoms in preventing the spread of AIDS. The gravity of the need for a concentrated national effort against the spread of AIDS was underscored not long afterward by a report from the prestigious National Academy of Sciences, which charged that the federal government's response to the AIDS epidemic had been dangerously inadequate. The report called for a $2 billion-per-year educational and research effort to avert what it called a "medical catastrophe." The academy requested the creation of a national commission on AIDS, and a large-scale campaign in the news media, in education, and by public-health groups to warn people explicitly to protect themselves from AIDS by avoiding unsafe sexual practices and sharing needles and syringes for injecting drugs.

Several new studies, at the University of Miami and at Montefiore Hospital in New York, indicated that the AIDS virus was as easily transmitted from women to men as from men to women, but that infection from a single exposure during vaginal intercourse was very low, about 1 percent. Among couples who engaged in repeated, unprotected intercourse over one to three years, the transmission rate was over 80 percent. Among those who used condoms, the transmission rate was slightly more than 15 percent. In New York, another set of figures from the AIDS program at Montefiore Hospital revealed that AIDS had become the leading cause of death for women twenty-five to twenty-nine years old in New York City, the second leading cause of death for women thirty to thirty-four, and the third leading cause of death for women fifteen to nineteen.

In December 1986, researchers at the National Institute of Allergy and Infectious Diseases in Bethesda, Maryland, discovered that the AIDS virus might be able to spread by infecting cells other than those of the immune system in the bloodstream. Test-tube experiments indicated that the virus can directly infect cells of the colon and rectum. This could mean that it spreads via anal intercourse even when there are no breaks in tissues. One reason the virus attacks these cells may be that they produce on their surface a molecule called CD-4, which is also found on the surface of the T-4 lymphocyte cells usually attacked by the AIDS virus.

By January 1987, 29,186 cases of AIDS had been reported in the United States; 16,054 of those victims had died.

In early February, Zaire ended its secretive stand on its massive AIDS epidemic, began to attack the disease openly, and instituted several programs to try to limit its spread. At the time, it was estimated that 5 to 8 percent of the adult population of the capital city of Kinshasa — at least 100,000 people — were infected with AIDS.

In late February the CDC sponsored a forum for more than 900 federal, state, local, and private health officials, to confront the many issues involved in AIDS testing in order to set policy for limiting the spread of the disease. The conference's goal was to address issues such as whether or not everyone who attends a clinic for sexually transmitted diseases or a drug treatment program should be given the AIDS antibody test, and whether all pregnant women, all people seeking marriage licenses, all infants admitted to hospitals, and all sex partners of people with the AIDS virus should have to take the test. The forum concluded that there was a need to widen AIDS testing, but that testing should remain voluntary rather than be made mandatory and should be accompanied by adequate counseling and strong safeguards to keep test results confidential.

In March, a Louis Harris & Associates poll of 227 scientists from all major areas of medicine and biomedical research, which included six Nobel prize laureates, resulted in the prediction that by the year 2000 more than a million Americans will have developed AIDS.

Around this time, the AIDS epidemic began to show itself quite clearly in Western Europe. Four thousand cases had been reported, and WHO estimated that between 500,000 and 1 million Western Europeans had already been infected by the virus. This led to predictions that between 50,000 and 300,000 Europeans would die from AIDS by 1992. Before the end of the month, the Reagan administration issued an official AIDS education plan calling for very specific information on AIDS to be made available to Americans, including recommendations on the use of condoms to prevent the spread of the disease.

As mid-1987 approached, 32,000 Americans had been diagnosed as having AIDS, and 60 percent of them had died. Everyone involved in combating the AIDS epidemic agreed that the lone effective weapon against the disease was preventing its spread, and efforts in many spheres were gaining momentum. Educational and public-health measures were accelerating, and in New York and New Jersey, teams of former drug addicts had been hired to roam the streets warning addicts to give up their habits or clean their needles and avoid sharing them. Despite tremendous controversy, condom ads aimed at the prevention of AIDS began to appear in many major magazines and on many TV stations. The majority of the nation's largest school systems had introduced new and sometimes controversial lessons to teach youngsters about avoiding the disease.

In April the 1988 presidential race began to pick up speed, and Vice-President George Bush, a Republican hopeful, quickly injected the AIDS issue into the campaign by calling for mandatory AIDS testing for all couples who apply for a marriage license.

And across the Atlantic, research showed that AIDS had begun to spread from its stronghold in Central Africa into populous and previously untouched West Africa — Nigeria, Ivory Coast, Ghana, Senegal, Gambia, and Togo — home to almost half of the continent's sub-Saharan population.

Treatment

Progress in the search for effective treatments for AIDS is completely entwined with the slowly expanding body of knowledge about the HTLV-III virus, its behavior, its reproduction, its different forms, its genetic structure, and its biochemistry. Every new discovery about the virus opens another door to possible ways it might be attacked, eradicated, slowed down, or its devastating effects diminished.

So far only one drug, AZT, which acts to interrupt a step in the virus's reproduction, has proved effective in any way. And AZT is not a cure. It does not eliminate the virus from the body. Rather, it inhibits its spread from cell to cell and seems to prolong the lives of some AIDS victims. Although this is better than no treatment at all, it is not terribly exciting. And it is only a first step. But considering that the AIDS virus is emerging as an increasingly complex organism with a widening repertoire of destructive characteristics, it is impressive that we've arrived at even narrowly effective AZT in so short a time.

The quest for drugs to treat AIDS began in earnest as soon as

HTLV-III virus was identified. By the summer of 1985, the FDA had approved nine drugs for experimental human testing. These included suramin, interferon alpha, phosphonoformate, ribavirin, Imreg-1, interleukin-2, isoprinisine, and two other compounds. An experimental French compound called HPA-23 received widespread publicity when the actor Rock Hudson revealed during the summer of 1985 that he had AIDS and went to Paris for HPA treatments. HPA-23, the chemical name of which is antimonium tungstate, was soon approved for testing in the United States.

Yet the process of finding and then testing these drugs is laborious and frustrating. One problem with many potential anti-AIDS drugs is their toxicity and their often debilitating side effects. HPA-23, for example, can cause damage to the liver and to cells necessary to clot blood. Another problem is that in order to ascertain a drug's effectiveness with any accuracy, tests must involve expensive and sophisticated techniques in statistics, pharmacology, and toxicology. The search for anti-AIDS drugs is further complicated by the fact that the disease has a long asymptomatic phase, which may require one type of treatment, if it should be treated at all, along with its early ARC phase and full-blown AIDS, which may require other treatments. In addition, it may be necessary that truly effective AIDS medications be able to be combined with cancer chemotherapy agents, because so many AIDS patients are so prone to cancers like Kaposi's sarcoma and lymphomas. Finally, it will be difficult to find one drug that will accomplish all the things necessary actually to cure AIDS: preventing the HTLV virus from reproducing, eliminating the virus from the body, and also restoring the suppressed immune system to normal functioning.

The search for AIDS treatments was further complicated in mid-1985 with the growth of evidence that the HTLV virus can infect cells in the brain and central nervous system, as well as cells of the immune system. In fact, doctors estimated that up to 30 percent of all AIDS patients show some symptoms of infection of the brain or spinal cord, and the accompanying symptoms of dementia, memory loss, difficulty in making decisions, partial paralysis, and loss of muscle control. The virus's ability to infect the brain means that a fully effective AIDS drug must meet not only the requirements described earlier, it must also be able to cross the blood-brain barrier, a chemical feature of the circulatory system that prevents many substances, including many drugs, from getting into the brain. If no way is found to send an anti-AIDS drug across the barrier, the brain of an AIDS victim could conceivably become a sanctuary for the virus, rendering ineffective any drug treatment that might eliminate the virus elsewhere in the body.

Around this time, two other factors emerged which looked as if they might make finding an anti-AIDS drug still more difficult. One was the discovery by a scientist at NIH that not all AIDS virus types are the same. He found that viruses isolated from five different patients were substantially different from one another, yet all were recognizable as HTLV-III, and all caused AIDS. It was not clear whether this meant that different subtypes might require different treatments. And other work at NIH indicated that viruses other than HTLV-III might play a critical triggering role in bringing on AIDS in those carrying the virus but not exhibiting any symptoms. In some cell cultures, many infected T-cells died. But others survived and appeared to be perfectly healthy, while still harboring the AIDS virus in a latent form. When these latent cells were treated with chemicals known to stimulate virus production, the dormant AIDS viruses emerged from their inactive state into virulent, cell-killing activity. If the virus behaves similarly in humans, this could mean that the million or more Americans who may have been infected by the AIDS virus but who have not come down with the disease could succumb if the dormant AIDS viruses in their immune system cells are stimulated by a second AIDS infection, or by infection by another virus. In other words, it may be true that in some, or even all, cases, AIDS is brought on when a second viral infection acts as a trigger. No one knows yet how this aspect of the disease will will affect the search for treatments.

Despite all these roadblocks, scientists were beginning to make some headway by the end of 1985. A program sponsored by the National Cancer Institute had screened about 150 compounds for possible effectiveness, a number of drugs had been found active against the virus in the test tube, and new knowledge about the virus's makeup had spurred optimism over possible drug designs. Some of the new drugs had already been experimentally tried on a few patients.

All efforts had focused on finding substances that would strike the AIDS virus at one of the vulnerable points in its life cycle. The stages in the cycle are the same for all viruses: a period when the virus, which is made up of a protein coat wrapped around genetic material (RNA in the case of HTLV-III, which is a retrovirus), is outside its target cell before infection; a point when the virus attaches to the target cell; a stage in which the virus then inserts its own genetic material into the infected cell; a phase in which retroviruses use a special enzyme called reverse transcriptase to subvert the target cell's reproduction by encoding their own genetic instructions into the cell's DNA; the period during which this subverted DNA reproduces new viruses inside the cell by replicating the alien genetic material; the subsequent assembly of the new viruses; and, finally, the escape of a new crop of viruses from the now-destroyed cell, so they can spread farther.

At that time, three drugs appeared most promising: amantadine, which is used against viral influenza A, and vidabarine and acyclovir, which are effective against the herpes virus. Amantadine seems to act by interrupting the second stage of the cycle, when the virus sheds its protecting coat to inject genetic material into the cell. The other two drugs seem to interfere with enzymes necessary to the virus. Other strategies researchers would like to try involve interfering with receptors on the cell surface where the virus attaches and disrupting the process of assembly of new viruses inside the cell.

But the most interesting target for researchers' efforts is the reverse transcriptase enzyme with which the virus translates its RNA genetic code into the DNA form necessary to subvert the cell's reproduction. Viruses are difficult to attack with drugs because the treatment often destroys the cell the virus inhabits. But since humans do not produce reverse transcriptase, it appears that drugs that could inactivate that enzyme would halt the virus infection without harming the normal cells. Of the five drugs then known to act against AIDS in test tubes by inactivating reverse transcriptase, two, suramin and AZT, looked most promising. Suramin had been used for years to treat tropical parasitic diseases, and AZT was scheduled to begin its first limited human trials soon.

In addition, a new drug called AL-721 had shown promise in test-tube experiments, halting AIDS virus infections apparently by disrupting the virus's protein coat. And human tests also began with a drug called ribavirin, already in use against other viral diseases. Ribavirin's action against viruses is not well understood.

Some thought was also given at this point to combining virus-killing drugs with natural immune stimulants like interferon and interleukin-2, which used alone had shown little promise against AIDS. But perhaps the most intriguing new pathway toward a treatment seemed to be opening up through improved understanding of the virus's genetic makeup. Researchers at Harvard had discovered that the HTLV-III virus has a special gene, called the transactivating transcriptional gene, or TAT gene, that plays a vital role in the virus's ability to subvert cells. A drug that interfered with that gene or its product might prove very effective against AIDS.

Work got under way on devising new means for carrying anti-AIDS drugs across the blood-brain barrier, to prevent the brain from becoming a sanctuary for AIDS viruses.

Within a month, experiments using AZT indicated that the drug was effective in keeping the AIDS virus from multiplying in humans, and that it also appeared to prevent further weight loss in fifteen subjects who were tested. Around the same time, researchers at the CDC reported that they had found the mechanism by which the AIDS virus recognizes T-cells and then binds to their surfaces. They demonstrated that an AIDS virus attack begins when a protein called GP-110 on the surface of the virus binds to a surface protein on a T-4 cell, like a key fitting into a lock. The isolation of this mechanism provided a new target for possible drugs, which might prevent AIDS infection by blocking this attachment, or halt its spread in people already infected.

Another important step was taken several weeks later, when a joint research team from the National Cancer Institute and a company called Bionetics Research, Inc., succeeded in identifying the exact form of the reverse transcriptase enzyme used by the AIDS virus in its reproduction, and in producing the enzyme in a pure form. This will allow researchers to test anti-AIDS drugs that deactivate the enzyme directly against the enzyme itself, rather than on infected cells. The current method involves many variables. Using the pure enzyme will enable direct measurements of the interactions between the drug and the enzyme.

A few weeks later, teams at Harvard and the NIH reported that they had used gene-splicing techniques to render the AIDS virus harmless in laboratory experiments. The researchers had snipped out the virus's TAT gene, which is the blueprint for producing a viral protein that makes invaded cells produce very large quantities of virus material. It was initially thought that removing the TAT gene would merely slow down the virus's reproduction. But without the gene, the virus was completely unable to reproduce. Since human cells do not have a gene similar to the TAT gene, the experiment suggested a new route toward developing drugs to fight AIDS. Any drug that could effectively neutralize that gene and render the AIDS virus harmless would probably not harm AIDS patients.

More encouraging results arrived from a study of AZT being conducted jointly by the National Cancer Institute and Duke University Medical Center. Patients in the study who had received the drug for about eight months showed improvements including fewer fevers, weight gain, improved appetite, and the disappearance of infections. The most important outcome was that it indicated a drug could help AIDS sufferers reconstitute at least part of their immune defenses. Hopes ran particularly high for AZT's longer-term effectiveness, because the drug can bypass the blood-brain barrier and enter the central nervous system to halt the spread of AIDS in infected brain cells.

As summer approached, researchers at the Harvard School of Public Health announced the discovery of yet another gene in the AIDS virus. This brought the number of known genes in the virus to seven, making HTLV-III the most complex retrovirus known. When the new gene, called the "art" gene, was deleted from AIDS viruses, the viruses could no longer produce an infection. The art gene appears to be the blueprint for the production of a small protein that acts as a key to unlock internal machinery in the virus that produces new viruses and delays the production of virus particles from being completed inside the host cell. Like the TAT gene, the art gene immediately became the target of research to find drugs that will treat AIDS by specifically inactivating it.

Yet despite encouraging discoveries, there were indications that the more that was learned about AIDS, the more complex and intimidating its treatment would become. At an international meeting on AIDS in Paris, it was announced that doctors treating AIDS patients were seeing marked changes in the frequency and types of cancers and other diseases afflicting their patients. More and more AIDS patients seemed to be suffering dementia and other neurological symptoms because of AIDS infecting their brains, for instance, and there were many more cases of intestinal salmonella infections and pneumonia caused by streptococcus and hemophilus influenza bacteria. It was noted that the incidence of Kaposi's sarcoma had declined in the United States, and that there were several documented cases of people who had become infected with the AIDS virus and then had shown a spontaneous remission of their infection.

These revelations only added to concerns that arose earlier in the year when Dr. Luc Montagnier at the Pasteur Institute in Paris had announced the discovery of a second AIDS-causing virus — named LAV 2 — during his joint work with Portuguese researchers in West Africa.

At the same meeting, researchers from the National Institute of Allergy and Infectious Disease disclosed that they had used a bone marrow transplant from an AIDS victim's healthy twin, along with an antiviral drug and transfusions of healthy lymphocytes, apparently to restore the patient's severely damaged immune system to normal health. The patient, who had suffered from weight loss, swollen lymph nodes, and Kaposi's sarcoma, had improved enough to return to work. After the therapy, the patient showed normal immune responses to several tests, and had a significantly increased level of T-4 lymphocytes. Two other patients who received the same combination therapy failed to improve. Scientists who conducted the test could not explain why the first patient responded so well and the others did not.

In June, the federal government announced it would provide $100 million to fourteen AIDS Treatment Evaluation Units for intensified testing of anti-AIDS drugs. The five drugs selected for the trials, which involved 3,000 of the nation's 10,000 living AIDS patients, were AZT, Foscarnet, HPA-23, ribavirin, and dideoxycytidine.

By September, this program showed results. The drug AZT, manufactured by the Burroughs Wellcome Company, was shown to be the most effective. Federal officials announced that AZT was the first drug to show effectiveness against AIDS. It had markedly improved the health of patients taking it for three- and six-month periods. Only one of a group of 145 getting the drug had died, while sixteen out of a group receiving placebos had died. Those taking the drug had fewer infections, and fewer AIDS-related problems. Thousands of people were promised access to the drug within ninety days.

It was emphasized that AZT, which can be made artificially or manufactured from genetic material in fish sperm, was not a cure for AIDS, and that its side effects, which could be severe and include suppression of bone marrow function and anemia, might preclude many AIDS victims from taking it. Only certain AIDS patients appeared to benefit from the drug. The first patients to get AZT had suffered a first attack of pneumocystis carinii pneumonia. This group was estimated to encompass a little over half of the nation's 11,000 to 12,000 surviving AIDS patients. At that point, researchers were reluctant to speculate about whether or not other AIDS patients, like children, those with Kaposi's sarcoma, and those suffering from neurological disorders, would derive similar benefits. One worry was that a substantial number of AIDS patients would simply not be able to afford AZT once it was marketed. The cost was expected to be from $8,000 to $10,000 per year for each patient.

AZT was originally synthesized in the early 1960s, as one of a group of drugs called deoxythymidines, which cancer researchers had hoped to use to replace nucleotide molecules in the DNA of cancer cells in order to impair the cells' runaway growth. The drug failed as a cancer treatment, but researchers began investigating its ability to disrupt the replication of genetic material as a possible way to stop the reproduction cycle of the AIDS virus. It turned out that AZT is able to block the virus's reproduction at the point where its reverse transcriptase enzyme translates its RNA genetic material into DNA that will go on to subvert an infected cell's DNA and make it produce more viruses.

In November, yet a third type of AIDS-causing virus was found infecting several West African AIDS patients in Sweden. The virus was designated SBL 6669 V-2.

Near the end of the year, scientists at the University of California at San Francisco announced that, in test-tube experiments, they had shown that human suppressor T-cells could inhibit duplication of the AIDS virus. They had taken blood samples from three healthy men who tested positive for the AIDS antibody, but who had no traces of the virus in their blood. When T-cells with a protein called CD-8, which includes suppressor T-cells, were removed from the blood samples, the AIDS virus began to grow in the samples. The researchers said this indicated the removed T-cells had been inhibiting virus production. When they added the CD-8 T-cells back into the samples, the duplication of the virus was inhibited again. The scientists said that this kind of spontaneous immune control of the virus could explain why so many people infected with the virus do not come down with AIDS. They also claimed the experiment supported their theory that the virus tends to cause AIDS only in people whose immune systems (including suppressor T-cells) have been severely weakened by chronic infection with another disease. Other experts on AIDS called the conclusions highly speculative. The researchers went on to suggest that their findings pointed toward a possible means of treatment, in which patients' suppressor T-cells would be removed from their blood, the cells' numbers would be built up outside the body with natural substances such as interleukin-2, and the cells would then be returned to the patient.

Not long afterward, researchers at the National Institute of Allergy and Infectious Diseases reported that they had found support for the theory that AIDS viruses lying dormant in cells could be stimulated into reproducing themselves by subsequent infection with other viruses. The experiments may help explain why some people infected with the AIDS virus remain asymptomatic for many years, and then suddenly go downhill. In test tubes, the AIDS virus was activated by exposure to several DNA viruses, including herpes simplex, adenovirus, which causes respiratory infections, herpes varicella zoster, which causes chicken pox, and JC virus, which causes degenerative neurological diseases.

In January 1987, the government announced the imminent licensing of another new experimental AIDS drug to be made by Hoffman–La Roche, Inc. The drug, dideoxycytidine (DDC), would be be tested by the National Cancer Institute on patients in advanced stages of AIDS. In the laboratory, the drug was found to halt the replication of the AIDS virus, to begin allowing the victim's immune system to reconstitute itself. In tests on animals, DDC was found to be slightly more effective against the virus, and slightly less toxic to the body than AZT. It works the same way AZT does, by crippling the reproductive stage at which reverse transcriptase creates DNA to subvert the host cell's genetic machinery.

Small steps forward like the testing of DDC were put into perspective by more new insights about the AIDS virus's tenacity, unpredictability, and complexity. A study done by the CDC and the San Francisco Health Department indicated that the longer one is infected with the AIDS virus without showing any symptoms, the higher the risk climbs that one will develop AIDS. The chances of developing full-blown AIDS seem to rise every year after the initial infection with the virus. The study results revealed that only 4 percent of people infected with the virus will develop AIDS within three years, but that 14 percent develop it within five years, and 36 percent develop the disease after seven years.

And an assessment of knowledge to date about the virus caused leading AIDS researchers to express a degree of marvel at the virus's extraordinary complexity, and its many abilities to attack cells and resist attempts to treat it. For instance, the AIDS virus is now known to have at least eight and perhaps more genes, while common animal retroviruses have only three. Besides being able to attack T-cells, brain cells, and perhaps the cells of the colon, it was recently found that the virus can also infect and destroy monocytes and macrophages, other cells in the immune system. And the virus can also cause the cells it infects to fuse with other cells, to create gigantic, abnormal aggregations of cells called syncytia. These huge conglomerates then operate as giant virus factories, producing huge amounts of the virus before they die. And other research has begun to suggest that the AIDS virus damages the immune system not only by killing T-cells, but also by making the cells produce a protein that itself diminishes the immune system's strength.

Still, efforts to test potential new anti-AIDS drugs were expanding rapidly, and it seemed that by the end of the year, thousands more AIDS victims would be in experimental drug-testing programs. The National Institute of Allergy and Infectious Diseases took a leading role in sponsoring the creation of research consortiums among government scientists, universities, and drug companies. Five had been started since the beginning of 1986, and twenty more were planned for 1987, with an additional twenty for 1988.

The spectrum of experimental drugs to combat AIDS had been narrowed somewhat. AZT and now DDC are the top candidates to date. Suramin and HPA-23 had been dismissed as ineffective after initial concentrated testing. Ribavirin is still being tested, although many experts have reservations about its effectiveness, as is interferon alpha, which is believed to attack the AIDS virus at the end of its reproductive cycle, when new viruses bud from the surface of an infected cell. AL-721 is also still being tested, along with a substance called peptide T, which acts similarly, by interfering with the virus's ability to attach itself to a target cell, and phosphonoformate (Foscarnet), which attacks the action of a key viral enzyme. Newer drugs are made up of artificially produced fragments of DNA that glue themselves to key segments of the virus's genetic blueprints and shut them down.

The pleas of anguished, dying patients and their supporters had led the FDA to establish special procedures to evaluate and approve potential AIDS drugs much faster than usual. And patient demands for the drugs were not blunted by repeated warnings that not all drugs would work for all people, and that the drugs tend to be extremely toxic and have devastating side effects. So desperate were AIDS sufferers that they had generated a national under-ground network of "guerrilla clinics" that disseminate information that helps people to try to treat themselves by taking doses of photographic chemicals, a soybean derivative, a substance found in Japanese mushrooms, and an herbal tea made from the bark of a Brazilian tree. There is even a recipe for a homemade approximation of the drug AL-721, which can be kept in the freezer and eaten on bread or mixed into juice. Medical professionals express skepticism about all these home remedies.

Near the end of March, a French scientist described a slightly more orthodox, but nevertheless fascinating AIDS therapy he was experimenting with. The treatment had been tried on two African AIDS victims who were critically ill and were said to have recovered enough to return to work, though they were still infected with the AIDS virus. The treatment, which resembled the process of vaccination, apparently involved removing white cells from the patients' blood and treating them in such a way that they developed "a coating of viral protein." The cells were then returned to the patient's bloodstream, where they apparently stimulated a renewal of white blood cells and reconstituted the immune system.

At the end of March, the FDA finally approved AZT for commercial distribution under the trade name Retrovir. Because of concern over the drug's side effects, its manufacturer, Burroughs Wellcome, planned to limit its distribution to selected groups of patients. There were also disappointments and setbacks. The federal government's testing programs for AIDS drugs were far behind schedule, and drug manufacturers wrestled with their financial and research priorities. And wider use of the drug ribavirin was curbed by the FDA because of challenges to the accuracy of the claims of its maker, ICN Pharmaceuticals of Costa Mesa, California, about the drug's effectiveness.

In April, a report published by the Whitehead Institute for Biomedical Research in Cambridge, Massachusetts, explained the mechanism by which other infections were believed to set off dormant AIDS viruses. The T-cells that are attacked by the AIDS virus, the report's authors said, produce a protein called NF kappa B. This protein is the one subverted by the AIDS virus in order to make the cell produce more AIDS viruses. But in healthy cells, NF kappa B appears to play a role in activating the cells against any new infection. Because of the dual role played by NF kappa B in normal immune responses and in being forced to produce AIDS viruses, activation of the protein by any infection might also cause it to start its cell reproducing dormant AIDS viruses within it.

But as always seems to be the case in the ongoing campaign to find treatments for AIDS, this disturbing finding was balanced a few days later by an announcement that scientists at the University of North Carolina at Chapel Hill had used genetic engineering techniques to insert the TAT gene from the AIDS virus, which controls the production of reverse transcriptase, into harmless *E. coli* bacteria. The researchers were able to use chemical switches to tell the bacteria to start and stop making the enzyme. The bacterium seemed to produce the enzyme using the exact process the AIDS virus uses. And this, the researchers said, would make it easier to test new drugs designed to improve upon AZT's action, disrupting the enzyme formation process at different stages.

Vaccine

Limiting the spread of AIDS and finding treatments for those already afflicted are desperately important goals. But the real prize in the battle against AIDS would be a vaccine. A vaccine could not only drastically diminish the spread of the disease, it would also hold out the hope of its complete eradication. If an infectious agent cannot proliferate from victim to victim, it cannot maintain its population. And if a vaccine is dispersed widely enough that it cuts the agent's population and spread below a critical level, theoretically, the agent will simply disappear. This is exactly what happened a decade ago to smallpox.

Unfortunately, the search for an AIDS vaccine may be the most complicated and frustrating of all the efforts against the virus. The virus is still so little understood that it is difficult to manipulate it and its protein and genetic components predictably to create potential vaccines. The nature of its infectiousness — which can manifest as murderous virulence, apparently harmless dormancy, or some nonfatal in-between stage — makes it a hard target for vaccine studies. The fact that the principle of vaccination entails stimulating the immune system to create antibodies to repel viral or bacterial invaders, and that the AIDS virus attacks and destroys this very process, adds yet another level of complexity. There is also the problem of ineffective antibodies. In all other cases, a vaccine is designed simply to induce the body to produce antibodies, which are known to protect against the infective agent. But in AIDS, antibodies apparently offer no protection against the disease. All AIDS patients have antibodies to the virus, and all of them eventually succumb to AIDS. Finally there is the problem of testing and eventually safe use of such a vaccine. Researchers recoil at the thought that they must, at least now, expose human subjects to a virus that they know is 100 percent fatal and, beyond some minimal reduction of symptoms, untreatable.

The extreme danger posed by the AIDS virus has caused most vaccine research to bypass one of the most basic approaches to the problem: using a weakened or killed form of the virus to elicit an antibody response that will then protect the person who has been vaccinated. The virus is simply too dangerous for this approach. Instead, efforts have focused on using genetic-engineering techniques to produce viral forms or fragments that will elicit a full-blown antibody reaction, without endangering the person who receives the vaccine.

The first real step in this direction came in the spring of 1986, when researchers used gene-splicing techniques to remove the TAT gene from AIDS viruses. This gene controls the production of a protein that substantially boosts an infected cell's production of new AIDS viruses. Removing the gene left AIDS viruses completely unable to reproduce. Researchers immediately recognized that these viruses might be valuable as a vaccine, since they would elicit antibodies that would protect against unaltered forms of the virus, but could not themselves infect cells. Such genetically inactivated viruses have been incorporated into vaccine research, but could never be used until it was satisfactorily proved that they were incapable of regaining their infectious power.

The next stride came when two research teams at NIH and at a subsidiary of the Bristol-Meyers Company remodeled the common and widely used vaccinia virus to carry a gene from the AIDS virus. Vaccinia is the virus used to make the vaccine that eradicated smallpox, by far the most widely used vaccine ever developed against human disease. The implanted AIDS gene is the blueprint for two surface proteins of the AIDS virus. One is involved in the process by which the virus attaches to its target cell. The other plays a role in the virus's structure. Experiments showed that mice and monkeys inoculated with the remodeled vaccinia virus formed antibodies to the AIDS virus, and cells inoculated with the vaccine reacted as if they had been invaded by the AIDS virus and produced antibodies. Two routes were suggested for the new vaccine. One simply involves using it directly as a vaccine. The other would involve using the remodeled virus as a factory to produce large amounts of the AIDS virus surface or envelope proteins that are produced by the implanted genes, and then using these proteins, actually partial representations of the surface of the AIDS virus, as a vaccine.

During the summer of 1986, researchers at Harvard and at Genentech, Inc., in California reported finding that a bit of the protein coat surrounding the AIDS virus could be used to make antibodies that neutralized the virus in test tubes. They also managed to produce the protein, called GP-130, in large quantities. Since it is only a fragment of the virus's coat, the researchers were convinced it could not cause AIDS, and would be a good potential vaccine that should be further tested in animals.

A next step was taken in December 1986, when researchers at the National Cancer Institute, the Repligen Corporation in Cambridge, Massachusetts, Centocor, Inc., in Malvern, Pennsylvania, and Duke University Medical School showed that another surface protein from the virus, called GP-120, spurred high levels of antibodies to the AIDS virus in test animals such as goats and rabbits. This indicated the protein's potential as a vaccine. The researchers said it could be cheaply mass-produced in a pure form by using genetically altered bacteria. They pointed out the need to duplicate the result in chimpanzees, which are the only animals other than humans that can get AIDS from the virus, and then prove that it protects from infection by the virus. The researchers also noted that since the AIDS virus mutates rapidly, a good vaccine would have to protect against many mutant forms of the virus. The protein segment GP-120, they said, seemed to contain an area that would remain stable through such mutations, so it would be able to act as such a multistrain vaccine.

Weeks later a joint French and Zairian team of scientists stunned AIDS researchers by announcing that they had begun the first human experiments with a form of immunization against AIDS. The experiment was conducted in Zaire on a small number of people already infected with the AIDS virus. The study represented a new form of vaccination aimed not at preventing uninfected people from being infected with AIDS, but at benefiting people already exposed to the virus but not yet afflicted with symptoms. The technique being used was intended to stimulate the body's immune system to produce a huge amount of immune system blood cells called killer lymphocytes. The hope was that these superabundant lymphocytes would prevent the dormant AIDS virus from developing into active AIDS. The experimenters, from the University of Kinshasa in Zaire and the University of Paris, were secretive about details of their work. But some medical sources believed that the biological substance injected into the subjects to trigger the lymphocyte production was made up of fragments of the AIDS virus's outer coat. To prove the safety of the experimental vaccine, Dr. Daniel Zagury, the leader of the French team, injected himself with it.

By January 1987, Dr. Anthony S. Fauci, coordinator of AIDS research at NIH, told the Senate Labor and Human Resources Committee that human tests for some AIDS vaccines might take place as early as the end of 1987 or the beginning of 1988. He said his confidence grew out of the fact that there were now so many approaches being explored to a vaccine that one or another of them would have to be ready for human tests soon. He also cautioned that no one should expect an AIDS vaccine to become widely available until well into the 1990s. Another AIDS researcher added that the vaccine would almost certainly be made up of protein fragments of the virus. He also argued that once the vaccine was perfected, the government should make vaccination compulsory for everyone, to avoid the kind of large-scale heterosexual epidemic of AIDS in Africa. Another AIDS expert noted that the best way to accomplish wholesale vaccination would be to give the vaccine to children.

Within three months, it appeared that Dr. Fauci's projections would pan out. Several vaccine test programs were nearing the point of moving to human tests, while experts continued to caution that the odds of a licensed AIDS vaccine in the immediate future were very slim.

Researchers were hopeful that a single vaccine could deliver two types of immune response. One is the standard vaccine outcome, antibodies to fight off the invading virus. The other is called cell-mediated immunity, and would result in a bolstering of immune defenses to battle the AIDS virus once it has entered the body, the effect the French/Zairian vaccine researchers were seeking. One estimate said that AIDS vaccine research already included hundreds of scientists in at least thirty institutes around the world.

Two American research teams had applied for permission to begin human vaccine trials. One, at George Washington University in Washington, D.C., had a vaccine called HPG-30, made from a synthesized version of a part of a protein called P-17 from the inner shell of the AIDS virus. Part of the protein is believed to protrude out to the virus's surface, and it is believed that this segment is what stimulates the production of antibodies. A P-17 vaccine has the advantage of being based on a core protein of the virus. These are thought to be more stable and less prone to mutation than strictly surface proteins, and so might generate antibodies that could repel more strains of the changing AIDS virus.

In addition, P-17 levels in the blood seem to decline as AIDS progresses, so it is hoped that the vaccine may have the added effect of preventing those already infected with the virus from becoming ill. It has also been suggested that a test for blood level of HPG-30 might thus be a more accurate measure of the extent of AIDS infection than current tests that measure only the presence of antibodies.

The other team that has requested permission to test its vaccine is with a Seattle biotechnology company called Oncogen. Its vaccine is prepared from genetically altered vaccinia virus, which has had two AIDS virus genes inserted into it. The genes will make the vaccinia virus produce two of the AIDS virus's surface proteins, GP-110 and GP-41, which should stimulate the body to produce antibodies.

Genentech in San Francisco is developing a vaccine made from fragments of an AIDS virus protein believed to be GP-120, and may apply for approval to test in humans by late 1987. And researchers at the Wistar Institute in Philadelphia are using what may be the most novel approach of all. It involves first injecting animals with an AIDS virus protein to stimulate antibody production. Then that antibody is injected into other animals to form a second antibody, called an anti-idiotype. This second antibody is then injected into animals to form yet a third antibody, which should be a mimic of the first antibody, but less likely to be contaminated by infective material, and so safer. This third antibody would be used as a vaccine.

Testing the vaccines on chimpanzees is viewed as the final step before testing them on humans. The effectiveness of the vaccine is then usually tested by challenging it, by trying to infect the animals with the disease in question. But although chimps will develop swollen lymph nodes because of the AIDS virus, they do not develop full-blown AIDS. This makes them less than ideal for the critical last step. Added to this is the fact that they are an endangered species and in short supply. All this means that there may be good reason to bypass the chimpanzee testing stage and go directly to vaccine experiments on humans.

This has been done before, with the vaccines for whooping cough, hemophilus influenza, and meningococcus, but AIDS is so dangerous that many sides of the question must be considered before such a decision is made. Further ethical questions cloud other future decisions. How can one determine if a vaccine is having a useful effect, if volunteers are taking precautions anyway to avoid infection with the virus? Should one purposely try to infect vaccine subjects with AIDS to challenge their immunity? Is it ethical to give placebos to half the vaccine test group, as in traditional experimental design, when doing this would cheat the subjects, who would probably be high-risk individuals or their spouses, of the possible real protection the experimental vaccine might give them?

And finally, if and when an effective AIDS vaccine is developed, who should get it?

HERPES

Several years before AIDS forced Americans to completely reevaluate their sex lives, the herpes epidemic changed the pattern of sexual behavior in the United States, throwing into reverse the sexual revolution that had been careering along full tilt for over a decade.

A sexually transmitted viral venereal disease, herpes was thought until recently to claim 20 million victims. New detection methods now indicate, however, that more that 40 million people — one-fourth or more of the adult population — carry the disease. The number of those infected rises every day, but the increase has apparently slowed as many people have begun to reexamine their sexual and dating habits, curtail the number of their liaisons, and choose their partners more carefully while taking strict precautions not to catch the virus from those who are infected.

Nevertheless, an estimated 300,000 to 500,000 new cases occur every year, and since herpes is incurable, the pool of infected individuals never shrinks but only grows, thereby constantly upping the odds that more and more people will become afflicted. Although it is often painful, herpes is rarely life-threatening to most adult sufferers. Right now all herpes research is focused on only one thing: relief — a vaccine; treatments to alleviate recurring outbreaks; a way to curtail the virus's transmission; and perhaps, some day, a cure.

Genital herpes or herpes simplex type 2 is a member of a family of the most common human viruses. Type 2 herpes causes painful blisters on and around the genitals and initially appeared to be able to live only on the lower part of the body. The blisters fill with fluid and break open, leaving painful sores that can last for weeks. Just before and during this period the virus "sheds" and can most easily be transmitted to an uninfected person by contact with his or her skin.

Nearly identical herpes simplex type 1 is responsible for the familiar cold sores many people often experience around the mouth. At one time herpes type 1 was believed to be able to survive only on or near the face. In rare instances, type 1 herpes can cause an eye infection called herpes keratitis that can lead to blindness, or a rare form of encephalitis that is often fatal.

With the increased popularity of oral sex, type 1 lesions now routinely appear around the genitals and type 2 lesions are found on the lips and mouth, and researchers believe that the subtle chemical differences between the two strains may be disappearing. This could lead to only one major type of venereal herpes virus before long.

All herpes viruses have an affinity for nerve cells. This includes the other three common herpes viruses: Epstein-Barr virus, which is responsible for infectious mononucleosis, or "kissing disease"; cytomegalovirus, which is harmless in adults but is one of the leading causes of birth defects in fetuses that are exposed to it; and herpes varicella zoster, which causes chicken pox in children and in adults a painful condition called shingles. The virus's affinity for nerve cells accounts for its incurability and its maddeningly recurrent behavior.

When herpes type 1 or 2 invades the skin during the first exposure, the virus's DNA enters skin cells and takes control of their protein synthesis, forcing the cell to become a herpes factory — producing hundreds of thousands of new viruses. These invade other cells, which in turn produce more viruses. This cellular destruction produces the herpes blister.

The body's antibodies to the virus eventually contain its spread, limiting blister size, but the immune system does not complete the job of destroying all the invaders. The virus's tough protein coat partially protects it from antibodies, and the virus migrates away from the blister site to the nerve cells, which it enters. It then begins its latency stage: it does not destroy the nerve cells but lies dormant in them, out of reach of the immune system's antibodies. Facial herpes hides in the trigeminal ganglion, which enervates the face, and genital herpes hibernates in the sacral ganglion, which enervates the lower body. The blisters and sores subside and everything appears to return to normal. That is, until the right stimulus intrudes.

In response to many stimuli — emotional stress, the change in hormone balance during menstruation, fever, common skin trauma like shaving, sunburn, or minor surgery — the viruses emerge from their nerve cells and create a new outbreak of blisters and a new episode of easy contagion. This episode will also pass; the viruses will retreat and lie dormant until the cycle occurs again and again for the rest of the sufferer's life. Most people average four or five outbreaks per year, but some severe cases have one per month.

Until recently, it appeared that herpes was spread only during these outbreaks by contact with the blisters. In mid-1986, however, a National Institutes of Health study revealed that herpes sufferers could spread the virus to their sexual partners even during the latency period, when they were experiencing no outbreak of symptoms. This disturbing discovery undermined the confidence of clinicians, researchers, and herpes sufferers and their partners that one could avoid spreading the disease simply by refraining from sex when the herpes victim showed visible symptoms. Subsequent studies resulted in a doubling of the number of herpes victims to 40 million. Some research indicates that the number of those infected may be as high as 50 million.

Research in the mid-1970s seemed to indicate that women with type 2 herpes had eight times the normal chance of developing cervical cancer. In the past few years, however, these fears have faded as evidence has accumulated implicating another virus. But the fact that a female herpes 2 victim stands a 50 percent chance of passing the infection on to her child during birth if the disease is active in her birth canal has spurred a prodigious effort to find new ways to deal with the disorder. One-third of herpes-infected newborns die, one-quarter suffer brain damage and severe retardation, and 6 percent suffer mild retardation. Obstetricians can look for open herpes lesions on the mother near the time of birth, and can inspect the birth canal during labor and perform a cesarean section if necessary to protect the infant. But to date, little progress has been made toward developing a fast, accurate test that can identify the herpes virus amid the many cervical secretions during labor and warn of the need for such measures.

The virus's dormancy behavior is the biggest roadblock to finding a cure. The virus can be killed when it is accessible during an outbreak of blisters, but there is no known way to send chemotherapy agents into the host nerve cells during the dormant phase without destroying the cells. To accomplish this, much needs to be learned about the virus's molecular state during dormancy. Test-tube experiments have shown that the natural antiviral agent interferon can be used to activate blood monocytes (immune system cells) to discriminate between herpes-infected cells and normal cells and attack the infected ones. Still, most researchers agree that there are no imminent breakthroughs on the horizon in terms of a cure.

There are also problems in developing a vaccine against herpes. The body has no problem forming antibodies against herpes; it simply cannot apply these to the vulnerable viruses for long enough to kill them all in the periods between latencies.

So far, most research efforts have yielded treatments that neither cure nor prevent herpes infections. Instead, they have produced chemicals that will kill the virus in the lesions during the shedding phase and thus speed healing, shorten the length of the attack, and perhaps reduce the chances of the virus's transmission, or drugs that seem to prevent the virus from establishing itself in skin lesions during the first exposure if they are applied as an ointment within twenty-four hours of exposure.

The first oral anti-herpes drug was ara-A, marketed as Vidarabine. Its use is limited to fighting the rare herpes encephalitis and herpes keratitis. Its side effects are unpleasant and it is useless against common herpes type 1 and type 2 and is also too dangerous for use in any but very risky circumstances. Another drug, called 2-deoxy-D-glucose, is still in experimental use only and has proved effective in interfering with the virus's ability to multiply.

The only effective oral antiherpes drug is an oral version of acyclovir, which was approved by the FDA in 1982 and marketed as Zorivax in early 1985. Used by patients during their first episode of herpes, before the virus enters its latency phase, the drug significantly reduces the duration of the lesions, seems to inhibit new lesion formation, and also seems to diminish other symptoms like pain and malaise. The drug does not, however, prevent the virus from entering its latency stage, nor does it prevent recurrent outbreaks.

It also appears that acyclovir-resistant strains of herpes have developed. Researchers fear that overuse of the drug on too many patients may force a wholesale mutation of herpes to these resistant strains.

Experimental drugs have shown promise in test-tube or animal work over the past few years, but are still far from being perfected. These include: ribavirin, made by the American firm Viratek, which blocks the virus's protein synthesis; isoprinosine, made in America by Newport Pharmaceuticals but not licensed for sale in the United States, which boosts certain immune system functions against herpes; BIOLF-62 ointment, which seems to prevent herpes lesions when applied to the skin within twenty-four hours after exposure; three drugs, called BVDU, FIAC, and FMAU, which are effective against Epstein-Barr virus and herpes varicella zoster and may have some application against type 1 and 2 viruses; cyclaradine, a chemical cousin of ara-A, which seems more effective in topical application and may inhibit recurrent episodes; ABPP, which clears lesions quickly and appears to block transmission of the virus if applied to the skin before contact; DHPG, which in oral form appears sixty-eight times more effective than acyclovir; gossypol, a cottonseed oil extract that, in cultures, appears to prevent infection if applied before introduction of herpes and to limit the spread of the virus if added after infection; and acetylpiridin thiosemicabazones, which are said to be 100 times more effective than acyclovir at stopping herpes lesions, but which cannot stop recurrent attacks.

Some loosely structured experimentation has been done by dermatologists and patients engaging in self-medication with a natural amino acid called L-lysine. One of the eight essential amino acids, L-lysine appears to reduce the frequency and severity of herpes outbreaks. The experimentation developed a diet plan high in L-lysine, which, if combined with a dietary reduction of the amino acid arginine, which the herpes virus is said to find essential for protein synthesis, is claimed to combat the disorder.

Work on a herpes vaccine is progressing, though slowly. A

team at the University of Birmingham in England is testing a vaccine made from the killed viruses of type 1 herpes. It is given to the spouses of herpes sufferers, known to be at risk of contracting the virus. The team reports a 100 percent rate of effectiveness after two years. A similar test of a different vaccine, made from a fragment of dead virus, is still under way in Seattle.

Genetic engineers at the Centers for Laboratories and Research in Albany, New York, tested yet another experimental vaccine and found it effective in mice. This vaccine was made by splicing a fragment of herpes type 1 DNA into the DNA of a vaccinia virus, the same microbe used by Dr. Edward Jenner to create the very first vaccine, against smallpox, nearly 200 years ago. A second step was taken in 1985 in a joint study by researchers at the National Institute for Dental Research and the National Institute of Allergy and Infectious Diseases. They demonstrated that a similar experimental vaccine protected mice against death from ordinarily lethal doses of herpes 1 virus, and also protected two-thirds of the animals against the development of latent infections. The vaccine also gave the animals significant protection against herpes type 2.

Another tack has been laser therapy, which one researcher has found vaporizes herpes lesions and speeds healing.

The lack of a quick diagnostic test for herpes is a major problem, especially in the case of pregnant women. Doctors must be able to tell quickly if a woman in labor has an active outbreak in her birth canal, and current cell-culture methods take from three to six days. The Genetic Systems Corporation, however, in 1983 developed a test that uses monoclonal antibodies and can give results in twenty minutes. The NIH also developed a test, claimed to be as accurate as tissue cultures, that gives results in twenty-four hours. Both have yet to come into widespread use.

Another troublesome factor is the almost total lack of understanding of exactly how the various stimulating factors cause the latent herpes virus to become active again. One of them, emotional stress, is now known to be manipulable, though. Some researchers and counselors of herpes victims have demonstrated that techniques of stress-reduction like meditation, yoga, biofeedback, and other types of calming methods can actually help reduce the frequency of recurrent outbreaks.

Herpes is not the only new venereal disease to reach epidemic proportions over the past few years. There has also been a remarkable surge in the number of cases of chlamydia, caused by the tiny bacterium *Chlamydia trachomatis.* Chlamydia is by far the most prevalent sexually transmitted disease in the United States. There are between three and 10 million new cases every year, against two million of gonorrhea and 500,000 of herpes.

Newborn infants can develop chlamydial eye infections from their passage through the birth canal of an infected mother, and 5 to 10 percent of pregnant women seen at prenatal clinics are found to have chlamydial infections. Sixteen to 18 percent of sexually active teenagers carry the infection. In the middle and upper classes where gonorrhea is well controlled, chlamydia is the major sexually transmitted disease.

Chlamydia infections are often silent and show no symptoms in men or women, leading to unwitting transmittal to sex partners. In most cases, though, symptoms in men include urethritis, an infection of the urinary tract, and sometimes a potentially sterilizing infection of the testes. Symptoms in women are similar and can include abdominal pain and discharge. Women are often left sterile by silent cases, and chlamydia is also the leading cause of pelvic inflammatory disease, which can lead to damage of the fallopian tubes, a major cause of female sterility.

Symptoms of chlamydia are often confused with gonorrhea and brushed aside as "nonspecific urethritis" when gonococcus fails to show up in tests. Unlike gonorrhea, chlamydia cannot be treated with penicillin, but requires antibiotics like tetracycline or erythromycin.

Until 1983, chlamydia's quick detection was hampered by the lack of a quick, inexpensive, easy-to-perform laboratory test. Last year, however, the Syva Company in California, a subsidiary of Syntex, began marketing a test called MicroTrak, which uses monoclonal antibodies to identify even small concentrations of chlamydia in about thirty minutes. The test is a great improvement over current methods, which take several days, and is reported to be more accurate. It requires special equipment, though, and is not yet widely available. Another rapid chlamydia test, called Chlamydiazyme, has been approved by the FDA but so far has not been marketed.

Now that chlamydia can be quickly identified and successfully treated, the major bar to its control is the lack of knowledge, on the part of victims and physicians, that the disease is so widespread and so dangerous. The last step required for dealing successfully with chlamydia is educational, not purely medical.

STROKE

A stroke occurs when one of the arteries supplying blood to the brain hemorrhages or is suddenly blocked, cutting off or catastrophically reducing the blood supply to the brain cells it nourishes. The result is swift and devastating. The blood-deprived cells die or are severely damaged, and the bodily functions they control are drastically reduced or altogether lost.

Strokes can be mild or severe, and their effects can range from partial paralysis of a limb or part of the face, to the immobilization of an entire side of the body. The outcome depends on the area of the brain involved and the degree of damage to it. Stroke victims may lose their voices and experience partial or total deafness or blindness. They often experience severe disorders of speech, memory, and language use when damage occurs to the areas of the brain that control these abilities. Damage in other zones of the brain can yield crippling personality changes. Often, the result of a stroke is death.

Three million Americans have survived strokes, but the disorder is the third leading cause of death in the United States, behind heart disease and cancer. Every year, 400,000 people suffer strokes and half of them die. Of the other 200,000, about one-third recover enough to resume most of their former activities, although only 10 percent of them are able to return to work. Half the survivors remain handicapped — paralyzed or otherwise — to a greater or lesser degree. Fifteen percent of stroke victims are so severely affected they must be institutionalized. It is estimated that strokes cost the U.S. economy up to $10 billion per year in lost earnings and medical expenses.

The best news about strokes is that their incidence is in a steep decline that extends back almost forty years. A 1979 study done by the Mayo Clinic revealed that stroke incidence had declined by 45 percent between 1945 and 1974. The drop cut across all age groups and both sexes, and the greatest decline was among the very elderly, eighty years old and older.

Initially, no one could offer a clear-cut explanation for the decline. But after the 1983 National Conference on High Blood Pressure Control announced that the death rate from stroke had declined by 42 percent between 1972 and 1983, and the American Heart Association noted in 1984 that the death rate had dropped 46 percent between 1968 and 1981, researchers finally agreed on the reasons for the falling incidence.

Prevailing opinion cites the increasingly widespread control of high blood pressure (hypertension) by diet, exercise, and medication as one major explanation for the decline in strokes. And this new gain in hypertension treatment is laid to the activities of the National High Blood Pressure Education Program, which operates through 150 national organizations, the health departments of all fifty states, and over 2,000 community groups. The movement aims to alert laymen and physicians to the dangers of hypertension and the importance of treating it. Its effectiveness is notable: in 1970, only half of those with hypertension knew it; by 1980, three-quarters were aware of their condition. In 1972, only 16.5 percent of hypertensives had their pressure controlled. By 1983, 34.1 percent did.

Uncontrolled high blood pressure greatly increases the risk of a hemorrhagic stroke, in which the blood vessels "blow out" or bleed, and it also promotes atherosclerosis and the formation of cholesterol-related fatty plaques on the inside walls of arteries. Plaques narrow the arteries and eventually close them or allow them to be blocked by blood clots in thrombotic strokes, or permit blood clots wandering through vessels to lodge in narrowed openings to cause what is called an embolic stroke. These last two types account for 78 percent of all strokes.

Other probable reasons for the decline are changes in diet toward lower-cholesterol foods, which are less likely to abet plaque formation; a decline in smoking (cigarette smokers are two or three times more likely than nonsmokers to suffer strokes); and a rise in Americans taking regular moderate exercise. Recent studies have also shown that men who drink heavily (thirty or more drinks per week) are four times more likely than nondrinkers to have a stroke, and Americans have generally begun to reduce their alcohol consumption in recent years. Since all of these factors also bear on heart disease, it is likely that the American Heart Association's campaign to educate people about how to prevent heart disease has significantly affected stroke incidence as well.

In addition, the past several years have seen many of the scattered facts about stroke coalesce into a comprehensive body of knowledge that is helping physicians spot potential stroke victims earlier and offer preventive treatment sooner, and is helping laymen to spot stroke or stroke-risk symptoms in themselves and their families. It was once thought, for instance, that stroke gave no warning signs, but it is now understood that four-fifths of all stroke victims display a prior symptom called transient ischemic attacks or TIAs. TIAs are actually tiny, temporary strokes resulting from transient loss of blood supply to part of the brain. TIAs usually last a few minutes, and the victim recovers completely within a day. TIAs can involve weakness, numbness in an arm, leg, hand, or the face; difficulty in swallowing, speaking, or understanding speech; vision disturbances or ringing in the ears; dizziness, clumsiness, or mild loss of balance; fainting, often with double vision; sudden headaches; transient changes in personality, such as irritability, impatience, or suspiciousness; or unexplained forgetfulness.

Once TIAs or other signs alert a stroke-risk patient, recently discovered preventive measures can be taken. Taking about four aspirin per day, for example, has been found to make blood platelets so "slippery" that the probability of stroke-inducing clots is markedly reduced.

Advances in surgery for stroke have been remarkable, though they have yet to evolve into a safe, standardized treatment. And last year, studies indicated that the two most common surgical procedures to prevent stroke might actually be of questionable value.

One operation, called carotid endarterectomy, has been

around since the 1950s and is performed on more than 100,000 Americans each year. It involves opening the carotid artery, which supplies blood to the head and is easily accessible in the neck, and removing any plaque buildup in it. The internal branch of the carotid supplies blood to the brain, and many strokes are the result of blockage in it. The surgery is routinely performed on patients who exhibit murmurs in the carotid artery, a symptom that suggests a blockage, but who have not had a TIA. In the fall of 1986, the latest in a series of reports critical of the procedure called it unnecessary. The study, which was done at the University of Toronto, indicated that patients who had not experienced a TIA ran a less than 2 percent risk of a disabling stroke, while 3 percent of patients who underwent this surgery died in the hospital, and that the surgery itself could lead to strokes in up to 15 percent of patients.

Successful surgery on other arteries that supply blood to the brain had to wait until the maturation of microsurgery techniques in the late 1970s, when the development of operating microscopes suitable for brain surgery and of tiny probes, hooks, clips, suture needles, and sutures finer than a human hair made it feasible to work on tiny cranial vessels.

The most common procedure, which was perfected in 1979, is the extra-cranial–intracranial bypass, or ECIC, in which a scalp artery is rerouted through an opening in the skull to bypass a blockage in a cranial vessel and restore blood flow to threatened or deprived brain tissue. Each year, 2,000 to 3,000 of these operations were done in the United States. Until late 1985, all studies had indicated that the operation could prevent stroke in patients with clear-cut TIA symptoms, avert a second stroke in those who had had one (and were therefore statistically likely to have more), and even restore lost brain and body function in some cases. Of known high-risk patients who had the procedure for a study, data indicated that 76 percent no longer had a blood insufficiency to the brain, and 94 percent did not have a stroke. Without the surgery, their odds of stroke would have been 50 percent.

But two years ago, an eight-year international study, larger than any conducted previously, and rigorously comparing results of the surgery with the results of exclusively medical and nonsurgical treatment, concluded that the surgery added no health benefits beyond what was achieved by good medical care. The report, based on research done by the National Institute of Neurological and Communicative Disorders and Stroke in Bethesda, Maryland, said the surgery did not in fact reduce the number of future strokes or deaths from stroke in patients who had it. Indeed, the surgical patients had a slightly higher incidence of stroke than the medical patients. Other research indicates that the surgery is of value mainly as a means of restoring function to people who have already lost it because of prior strokes.

Unfortunately, surgery to remove obstructions from the many cranial arteries buried deep at the base of the brain remains extremely difficult and often impossible, despite microsurgery advances.

New diagnostic techniques have improved physicians' ability to ascertain what type of stroke a patient has suffered, so the proper treatment can be prescribed. CAT scans reveal whether a stroke was caused by blockage or hemorrhage, and PET scans trace the extent of diminished brain-cell activity. The most exciting diagnostic breakthrough, however, may come from a system that appears to be able to reveal stroke risk long before the danger point is reached.

The new device was invented by pathologist Gene Bond of the Bowman Gray School of Medicine in Winston-Salem, North Carolina. It uses ultrasound emissions to detect plaque buildup in the carotid artery without breaking the skin, injecting radioactive dyes, or exposing the patient to X rays. It sends sound waves through tissues and receives the waves as they bounce back, forming a reflected visual image of the structures in much the same way radar uses radio emissions. The device enables the physician to monitor not only the blood channel inside the artery, but also the slightest beginnings of plaque buildup, down to layers only one sixty-fourth of an inch thick. In the past it was possible to detect plaque only after it had built up to dangerous levels, critically narrowing the artery. This method allows early enough detection so the patient can change dietary habits and perhaps avoid further damage.

The device must be clinically tested before is becomes commercially available.

Advances have come slowly in the area of therapy for stroke victims, but over the past few years, they have begun to mount. Lasers and balloons inserted into clogged arteries can dissolve some clots. A medical team at Umea University Hospital in Umea, Sweden, two years ago began treating stroke victims by thickening their blood by draining part of their whole blood and replacing it with dextran, a blood substitute. This causes the brain to carry away the fluid that normally collects around injured cells, reducing swelling and allowing nutrients to flow to the damaged area. The treatment significantly shortened the hospital time of the patients and dramatically boosted their recovery. An American research team successfully tested an opposite approach, thinning the blood to let it slip past the blockage to nourish damaged tissues. Both techniques work best with patients who have suffered the least serious strokes.

Little can be done to restore function to brain cells long dead because of blood loss. But a 1982 study at the University of Michigan indicated that some reversal of paralysis through reengorging undersupplied brain tissues can be achieved with a novel application of a very old method: blood transfusions. Transfusions increase the heart's output of blood, and it is thought that this increased output is responsible for boosting the blood supply to stroke-deprived areas of the brain. The Michigan team also noted that high-stroke-risk patients with atherosclerosis or hypertension often show a decrease in blood volume because of dehydration, and that this decrease in volume sometimes seems to be the precipitating factor in their strokes. Reversing this state with increased blood flow via transfusions seems to reverse stroke effects in some cases.

Perhaps the most dramatic new stroke treatment is still highly experimental. Developed at Thomas Jefferson University, it uses the cerebrospinal fluid that bathes the brain to deliver a highly elevated dose of oxygen directly to the damaged, oxygen-deprived cells. This is done by injecting into the spinal fluid a fluorocarbon oil called perfluorobutyltetrahydrofuran, which carries almost half again as much oxygen as blood. The fluid carries so much pure oxygen that rats submerged in it for hours can survive just by breathing it. In laboratory experiments on animals, the Thomas Jefferson University team used the technique to resuscitate animals that were brain dead after massive strokes. Bathed in the oxygen and nutrient-rich fluid, the brain seems to restart cells the stroke had shut off. The brain begins absorbing its nutrient fuel, glucose, almost immediately, and the level of lactic acid, a waste product, drops. Brain-dead animals treated this way were able to sit up and act normally after twenty-four hours. The researchers predict that the treatment, which has yet to be tried on humans, should be effective, provided it is begun within three or four hours after a stroke and continued for four or five days while doctors restore normal blood circulation with drugs or surgery.

Despite breakthroughs just over the horizon, the major treatment for stroke victims is still physical therapy to encourage the return of motor, speech, and other lost abilities. But even this area has some new wrinkles. It has recently been understood, for instance, that physiotherapy is far more effective than once believed if it is started immediately after the stroke, before muscles atrophy and joints stiffen, and is intensively continued, often to the point of exhaustion and frustration, for an extended period, often for years.

Intensive speech-therapy programs are also showing dramatic results. Biofeedback is being used to improve physiotherapy. And rehabilitation centers, which are increasing in number, are adopting a coordinated team approach that bombards the stroke patient with experts in each of his areas of need. A typical team includes a psychiatrist, a physical therapist, a speech therapist, an occupational therapist, a recreational therapist, and a social worker.

It is also now understood that stroke victims often fall prey to serious depression that impedes their improvement, so quick, intensive psychotherapy is a new part of the rehabilitation regimen.

The last few years have also seen a rise in so-called stroke clubs, community organizations made up of stroke victims and their families. These groups provide emotional support and advice for the relatives of stroke victims who are trying to cope with the burden of caring for a disabled loved one. And they often have day-care programs where stroke victims can mingle with others with the same problem, to overcome the isolation that often accompanies their condition, and participate in recreational activities that enhance their recovery.

Most experts agree that because physical therapies are the only real treatment for stroke, the most significant factor in a patient's recovery is sheer will, dogged determination on his part and on the part of family members who help him.

AGING

Perhaps the greatest breakthrough in the treatment of age-related disorders has been conceptual and not strictly medical: many conditions long believed to be an inevitable part of the natural process of aging — progressive debility, senility, extreme physical fragility, loss of the ability to care for oneself — have recently been recognized as distinct diseases or the result of disease processes. Many of them, it is known, can be treated, prevented, or alleviated.

There is also a new understanding of the important effects that social factors, like isolation and a diminished ability to get around, can have on the health of older people, and also of the role played by psychological states like depression in the medical condition of the elderly.

Many of these gains stem from accelerating research in all areas of gerontology, the study of aging, and geriatrics, the medical specialty that deals with older people. Much of the impetus for this work comes from the National Institute on Aging (NIA), which was formed in 1976. The formation of the NIA was an answer to the statistics on the present and future demographics of American society: people over sixty-five now number 23 million, about 11 percent of the population. They account, however, for 29 percent of the national bill for health costs. By the year 2020, there will be 43 million citizens age sixty-five and older.

Although 80 to 90 percent of the elderly describe their health as good to excellent, medical problems take a terrible toll among older people. This is especially true because of the widespread lack of knowledge among not only the elderly and their families, but also among physicians, about the specialized symptoms older people exhibit when suffering from common diseases. For example, heart attack, hypoglycemia (low blood sugar), infections, malnutrition, hyperthyroidism, kidney failure, and vitamin deficiency all have clear symptoms in someone fifty years old. In someone much older, their only sign might be a mental confusion. Many older people misuse their drugs, taking too much or too little because they cannot read instructions on pharmacy labels, or because bottles are too difficult to open, or because they mix their prescription drugs with over-the-counter medications and cause adverse reactions. Many elderly people suffer from drug intoxication as well. Dosages change radically with advanced age, but many doctors don't know this and overmedicate their elderly patients. Many elderly suffer from the effects of drug interaction from multiple medications, and appear to be ill or mentally confused.

This often leads to a misdiagnosis of the aged person's problem, which is frequently seen as senility. This, in turn, leads to unnecessary institutionalization or failure to treat the actual disease, both with predictably negative results.

Most of the medical profession has been slow to take up this specialized geriatric knowledge. There is also a critical shortage of geriatricians to treat the elderly, recognize their special symptoms, and render proper care. As of 1981, there were only 600 geriatricians out of a physician population of 250,000, and only forty of them were qualified enough to teach the specialty to other doctors. By 1986, there were between 300 and 400 qualified to teach, still far short of the goal of 1,300 physician instructors nationally. There is, however, an increasing interest in the field among medical schools and medical students: eighty-one of 126 medical schools now offer at least some geriatrics courses, and Harvard, Johns Hopkins, Mount Sinai, and UCLA medical schools have full-fledged geriatric programs. But America will need 9,000 geriatricians by 1990, and it will have only 800.

The greatest barrier to the successful spread of new knowledge about the medical problems of the aged is the entrenched body of stereotypes and myths about how people act and feel when they get old. The faster physicians, the elderly, and the families of the aged can break through these misconceptions, the more quickly care for the elderly will improve.

Standing out from the medical profession's growing ability to differentiate between the signs of normal aging and the symptoms of disease are several issues that tend to overwhelm almost everything else going on in the field: Alzheimer's disease, or senile dementia, the most dramatic and frightening; osteoporosis, which causes profound weakening of the bones and leads to falls and injuries; and nutrition and its importance in the health of the elderly and its role in prolonging life.

Alzheimer's Disease

Until around 1977 senility — the progressive loss of mental facilities, deepening confusion, loss of ability to care for oneself, irrational behavior — was seen as an inevitable consequence of aging for many. But about seven years ago, the medical community finally recognized a body of work that had been growing for years and acknowledged that this was not so. It turns out that only 10 percent of people over sixty-five have any organic brain conditions underlying apparent senility, and that three-quarters of these people have Alzheimer's disease. The remaining quarter largely suffer from multiple infarct brain damage from an accretion of small strokes. Everyone else who appears senile is usually suffering from another medical problem like overmedication or hypothermia (abnormally low body temperature) that mimics senility until properly diagnosed.

Between 1.5 and 2.5 million Americans suffer from Alzheimer's disease. The cause of the disease is unknown, there is no known treatment, and the condition is considered incurable and irreversible.

Alzheimer's is extremely hard to diagnose in its early stages because it often begins with a pattern of recent memory loss that resembles the innocuous and normal memory decline that comes with aging. But Alzheimer's rapidly progresses to an inability to calculate figures, a growing disorientation, a constant state of agitation, and shorter and shorter periods of memory retention, often only a few minutes. The victim's condition rapidly deteriorates to include hallucinations, personality changes, irrationally angry and violent behavior, and ultimately leads to a loss of any ability to care for oneself, incontinence, and finally death.

Some people live for over a decade with the disease; some die within a few years. An estimated 100,000 to 200,000 deaths per year are attributed to Alzheimer's disease. Families are devastated by the toll of caring for these patients, and such hard-to-handle individuals are often impossible to place in custodial care.

An Alzheimer's victim's brain undergoes gross physical changes. The brain is shot through with lesions called neurofibrillary tangles and others called neuritic plaques. The tangles are fibrous masses found in damaged brain cells. The plaques are dead spherical masses believed to be the corpses of destroyed brain cells. Recent work shows that there is a direct relationship between the number of plaques and the degree of dementia: the more plaques, the more demented the patient. Nothing else is known about this correlation.

Other recent work has revealed that Alzheimer's involves a deficiency in the neurotransmitter acetylcholine, which conducts messages between brain cells. And it is now known that much of the cell destruction in the disease takes place in a specific area of the brain called the hippocampus, which is concerned with creating and cataloging memories. A nearby area called the nucleus basalis of Maynert is also affected: one researcher found that one victim had lost 90 percent of certain cells in this area.

PET scans have shown that Alzheimer's-afflicted brains are very deficient in their ability to use glucose, which is the energy source for neurons. This defect shows up most markedly in the posterior parietal lobe of the brain, or "association cortex," which integrates sensory input. It seems, then, that there is chemically more to Alzheimer's than just an acetylcholine deficit. And no one knows if the glucose and acetylcholine pathologies are causes or symptoms of the disease.

There have also been recent findings of elevated levels of aluminum in the neurofibrillary tangles, leading to the notion that accumulated toxins may play a role in the disease. One study has indicated that smoking a pack of cigarettes or more per day quadruples the risk of developing Alzheimer's. Other work indicates that Alzheimer's runs in families and that this hereditary form of the disease may account for up to 10 percent of Alzheimer's cases. The location of a gene that may be linked to conferring susceptibility to Alzheimer's, on a chromosome near a gene known to control immune system functions, implies that Alzheimer's may be linked to a malfunction of the brain's immune system.

New findings using the reactivated DNA and RNA molecules from the frozen brains of deceased Alzheimer's victims indicate that brains affected with Alzheimer's produce a drastically reduced amount of protein, about half the normal level. Again, it is not known if this deficit is a cause or a symptom of the disease.

Theories about the cause of the disease include a slow virus, which is communicable, takes decades to begin its damage, and is specific to acetylcholine-producing cells. The infectious virus theory is supported by some evidence that brain cells initially try to defend themselves against the disease's damage by sprouting new intercellular connections, before they are overcome. Another possible culprit could be prions, extremely primitive infectious agents even less sophisticated than viruses. One researcher thinks he has found prions in the brain waste product amyloid, found in neuritic plaques of Alzheimer's victims.

Research on Alzheimer's disease has been difficult, because it is hard to diagnose in its early stages; it is also difficult to chart the course of its full progression. Ethical constraints impede taking brain biopsies from living Alzheimer's sufferers to make a diagnosis: there is no precedent for such invasive procedures that offer no therapeutic benefit to the patient, while posing potentially serious complications. Work is under way to find practical diagnostic tests. The most recent advance was the discovery last year, by researchers at Albert Einstein College of Medicine in the Bronx, of a protein, designated A-68, which was found only in the brains of Alzheimer's patients, and only in the regions of the brain affected by Alzheimer's. The protein was also found in cells that had not yet been observably damaged by the disease process, indicating that it appears very early in the disease and may even be a causative factor. Months later, the same team found that the protein was detectable in spinal fluid, meaning it could be used as a marker to diagnose the disease. However, the test is still impractical and highly experimental, and many questions about the meaning of its findings probably won't be answered for several years.

Research has also been hampered because no animals spontaneously develop any disease similar to Alzheimer's. This has meant there has been no animal model on which to conduct experiments, but this may soon change. In late 1986, research teams at Johns Hopkins Medical School and the University of California at San Francisco reported developing new strains of laboratory animals that are susceptible to Down's syndrome. Down's syndrome is a genetic disorder that produces mental retardation. It is linked to an abnormality in the twenty-first chromosome. As people with Down's syndrome age, their brains develop the same cellular changes that occur in Alzheimer's victims. There appears to be some link, as yet not understood, between the processes of Alzheimer's disease and these changes in the brains of those with Down's syndrome, and Down's syndrome victims are being studied for clues that might expand the understanding of Alzheimer's. Animals that can be given Down's syndrome will help this along, and may even be the first step toward future strains of laboratory animals that can be given Alzheimer's disease.

Not surprisingly, the most encouraging recent strides toward unraveling Alzheimer's disease came with several discoveries in early 1987 about the role played in the disease by genes located on chromosome 21. One such gene was isolated almost simultaneously by laboratory teams in New York, North Carolina, and Boston. The gene appears to be responsible for making a large protein that is the precursor to smaller proteins making up the amyloids that form plaques and tangles in brain cells damaged by Alzheimer's. At the same time, a research team at Massachusetts General Hospital found strong evidence that a defective gene on chromosome 21 causes familial Alzheimer's disease, which is passed from generation to generation. It is still unclear whether the defective gene in the hereditary form of the disease is separate from the gene that controls production of the preamyloid protein, or if the research teams are all studying the same gene.

A few weeks later, another group of researchers reported finding an abnormal duplication of the amyloid-producing gene in several Alzheimer's patients and in two patients with Down's syndrome. The Alzheimer's patients were sporadic cases of the disease, not cases of hereditary Alzheimer's, indicating that the genetic component of Alzheimer's was not linked solely to the familial form of the illness. The finding of a parallel genetic flaw in a Down's syndrome sufferer strengthened the link between the two conditions.

These breakthroughs bolster the view that there is a powerful genetic component in Alzheimer's disease. Yet scientists still do not know why the patients have the extra copy of the gene, what role is played by environmental stress, or even whether the amyloid plaques and tangles moderated by the gene are a cause of Alzheimer's disease or merely the products of cell breakdown because of it.

Work also proceeds on treatment and cure. Drugs called aminopyridines are being experimentally given to patients to increase the calcium uptake of their brain cells. Depressed calcium absorption leads to an acetylcholine deficit, and the calcium uptake problem is associated with Alzheimer's, as is acetylcholine shortage. Enzyme-replacement therapy is being tried, in which patients are given elevated levels of choline in their diet, in the hope that this chemical precursor to acetylcholine will somehow boost the neurotransmitter deficit. Marked improvement in patient behavior was observed for periods after recent experiments in which patients were given the opiate antagonist naloxone, which blocks the action of endorphins, naturally produced opiate-like substances. One radical experiment involved infusing bethanechol chloride, which is similar in action to acetylcholine, directly into the brains of Alzheimer's victims, and showed some tentatively positive results.

The latest advance has come from studies with an experimental drug called tetrahydroaminoacridine, or THA. Researchers at two California hospitals reported that THA significantly improved the memories of twelve people, and temporarily reduced their Alzheimer's symptoms. One woman was able to resume cooking, cleaning, and homemaking tasks, another patient was able to return to work part-time, and a third person was able to play golf each day. The drug seemed to have no serious side effects. When the patients stopped taking THA, their symptoms returned, and the research team noted that it was expected that THA would lose its effectiveness with Alzheimer's victims as their disease progressed. Other researchers responded coolly to the findings, because earlier studies of THA did not yield such dramatic results and because the more severely affected patients responded least well to the drug.

The greatest hope for a future treatment for Alzheimer's may be found in a technique for transplanting healthy, acetylcholine-producing cells into the brains of victims. Experiments with monkeys show that the brain's "immunologically privileged" status allows such cells to continue to produce the acetylcholine, while they are not rejected as forcefully as they would be elsewhere in the body. The animals that received the cells regained a significant percentage of memory function that was lost when their acetylcholine-producing cells were experimentally destroyed.

For now, Alzheimer's disease remains unstoppably progressive. The National Alzheimer's Disease and Related Ailments Association supports a growing network of family support groups to help victims' loved ones deal with the strain of caring for them. Some of the programs offer day care so the patients can leave the house and engage in recreational therapy. This seems to make the disease's progressive ravages easier for everyone to bear, at least for a while. Beyond this, there is simply nothing to be done.

Osteoporosis

The recognition of this disease put to rest the notion that extreme frailty and broken bones come along with aging.

It turns out that many of the fractures suffered by the elderly are the result of drastically weakened bones that have lost an abnormally large amount of calcium because of osteoporosis. The condition is more prevalent in women than in men and may be responsible for 600,000 fractures per year among the elderly, including 190,000 hip fractures that often lead to complications ending in death.

Bone is not static but is constantly changing, undergoing alternate cycles of resorption (dissolution, in which calcium is freed into the blood and body fluids) and formation, in which new bone is laid down. It is believed that when calcium levels elsewhere in the body decrease, resorption occurs in order to maintain a balance of the mineral. Resorption and formation normally balance each other out so that an adult's bone calcium level remains constant.

Osteoporosis results when the balance between these two processes is disrupted, there is more resorption than formation, and the bones lose calcium and are weakened. One bar to further advances in treating this problem is that the mechanisms of this cycle are poorly understood. It is now known that postmenopausal women are predisposed to osteoporosis and that their loss of the hormone estrogen is the single most powerful factor in their bone loss. This process can be exacerbated by cigarette smoking, heavy alcohol consumption, lack of physical activity, and long-term treatment with corticosteroid drugs.

Research has shown that contrary to popular belief, calcium requirements go up in old age, not down. This knowledge has led to some techniques for slowing calcium loss in osteoporosis victims, including ingesting 1,500 milligrams of calcium per day in foods such as skim milk, or in the form of readily absorbable dietary supplements. Some researchers dispute the value of calcium supplements, reporting that in postmenopausal women, calcium supplements of up to 2,000 milligrams per day fail to affect rapid bone loss. As yet there is no known way to restore calcium and strength to bones already weakened by the disease. And regular, vigorous exercise is the only known way to increase bone mass after bone stops growing at maturity.

Estrogen-replacement therapy, or ERT, in which sufferers are given the hormone when they stop producing it after menopause, dramatically slows calcium loss and has been used for ten years. At one time, 20 million women received ERT. But some years ago, their numbers dropped when it appeared that long-term use of estrogen was linked to increased rates of uterine cancer, and most doctors stopped writing prescriptions for the drug. However, more recent research indicates that the cancer risk was greatly inflated, and that any remaining risk can be dramatically reduced or completely eliminated if ERT is given in a rotating three-week cycle, in combination with the hormone progesterone. Screening tests before beginning ERT can also eliminate women at high risk for developing cancer. Despite side effects, like increased risk of gall bladder disease, high blood pressure, blood clots, and abnormal vaginal bleeding, new forms of oral estrogen and skin-patch administration of low doses of the hormone have led to a resurgence in the use of ERT. The therapy is usually administered in conjunction with calcium supplements and a program of vigorous physical exercise.

Other types of therapy are being tried, and none of them is yet out of the stage of clinical trials.

Calcitonin, a thyroid hormone, and stanolozol, which is derived from male sex hormones, both show promise in slowing bone loss and increasing bone mass. A vitamin D derivative called 1,25-(OH)2D increases the absorption of calcium by the digestive tract (this absorption tends to fall off in old age) and seems to slow osteoporotic bone loss. Clomiphene citrate, an antiestrogenic agent that at high doses mimics the effect of estrogen, is being tried as a replacement for ERT. Researchers have found it to be more effective than ERT, with a lower cancer risk. Some researchers believe that in the near future, it may be possible to treat or reverse osteoporosis by using substances called skeletal growth factors and other body chemicals that affect bone growth, such as prostaglandins and cytokines. Preliminary studies at Massachusetts General Hospital indicate that parathyroid hormone administered together with vitamin D can increase the formation of bone lost in the vertebrae.

Recently, previously unknown bone proteins and other body substances that seem to control the buildup and breakdown of bone have been discovered, and some researchers envision using them in the future to prevent and treat osteoporosis.

A new CAT scan technique shows promise in measuring the bone loss in spinal vertebrae of women with the disorder, allowing prompt treatment to avoid painful spontaneous "crush fractures" of the backbone. Administration of a kidney hormone called calcitrol, which increases bone mass with minimal side effects, seems to help the condition.

The most controversial new therapy involves treatment with fluoride combined with calcium supplements. This does increase bone mass, but there is argument over whether the improved bone is actually stronger. There are also some unpleasant side effects, which have led some researchers to warn against this therapy.

One problem with osteoporosis has been the lack of a good means for early diagnosis so preventive measures can be taken before bone weakening progresses too far. A new, experimental test, which has been used on monkeys, may solve this problem by the early 1990s, if upcoming human studies pan out. The test involves administering a hormone antagonist, which briefly simulates the conditions of menopause under which rapid bone loss begins. Urine calcium levels are then measured over ten days, before and after the antagonist was given, to ascertain the subject's possible rate of future bone loss, and consequent susceptibility to osteoporosis.

Much emphasis is put on the prevention of osteoporosis. This involves increasing daily calcium consumption from the normal level of 800 milligrams per day to 1,500 milligrams per day and avoiding inactivity, which leads to bone loss. Increased calcium consumption can also slow bone loss in people who have already developed the disease.

Nutrition

Diet has turned out to be one of the most critical factors in the medical well-being of the aged. Scientists estimate that anywhere from 15 percent to 50 percent of Americans over the age of sixty-five consume too few calories, vitamins, and minerals for good health.

Older people, especially those who live alone, have a tendency to become malnourished. Factors like loneliness after the loss of a spouse, depression, reduced physical abilities, dental problems, arthritis, failing eyesight, and age-diminished senses of smell and taste all work against older people's shopping adequately, preparing, and eating a balanced diet. Also, certain prescription drugs can interfere with the digestive system's absorption of vitamins and minerals.

The widespread impact of this tendency toward inadequate nutrition has only recently been recognized. The myth that food requirements decline as one ages predominated for a long time. In fact, *caloric* needs are reduced with age but *nutritional* requirements remain the same. Symptoms induced by malnutrition can mimic senility and lead to misdiagnosis and can exacerbate existing conditions like type II diabetes. Recent findings indicate that malnourishment may cause a good part of the decline in the effectiveness of the immune system seen in the elderly. This diminished disease resistance used to be thought of as a natural part of the aging process. But experiments have now shown that nutritional supplements can partly restore the flagging immune systems of malnourished elderly patients.

The need for adequate nutrition among the elderly has been addressed by federally funded hot-meal delivery programs at senior centers for those who can go out. In fact, these congregate eating programs have evolved to serve medical, social, and psychological functions as well. The regular gathering with peers works against isolation and depression and fosters involvement with recreational activities. The gatherings are used to bring important health information to the participants, like education programs concerning nutrition and medical issues. The programs also function as portals to offer access to out-patient nursing and medical and monitoring care.

Another breakthrough concerning the role of nutrition and aging comes out of the work of Dr. Raymond Walford, author of the book *Maximum Life Span.* Walford advocates "undernutrition without malnutrition" — caloric intake that is consistently 40 percent lower than that required for so-called normal body weight. His research shows that if an eating pattern like this is established early in life, it may retard many of the functional biological declines associated with aging. Animal experiments indicate this is true for cancer, kidney disorders, and some autoimmune diseases.

Walford claims that even if started late in life the regimen can increase longevity, perhaps from the current upper limit of 120 years to 140 years. He notes that in cultures with high populations of healthy old people, individuals consume less than 1,500 calories per day and tend to be small (about five feet three) and slight (about 100 pounds).

Moderate exercise is also accepted to retard normal age-related declines like high blood pressure, hypoglycemia, arthritis, osteoporosis, elevated cholesterol, and depression, and has been demonstrated to literally add years to one's life. Research now indicates that up to 50 percent of the functional declines associated with aging are the result of disuse and can be reversed by exercise.

Other recent insights into the proper medical care of the aged comes from the discovery that hypothermia, or abnormally lowered body temperature, is a hidden medical problem for many elderly. It can affect people indoors when the temperature is 65 degrees or less, or can result from thyroid or pituitary malfunction, or from phenothiozine tranquilizers, which are often prescribed for the elderly. The condition's symptoms include clumsiness, altered gait, poor coordination, stiffness, depressed central nervous system function, slurred speech, pneumonia, heart failure, stroke, coma, and death. It is often misdiagnosed.

Hypothermia can be avoided by wearing warm clothes and carefully monitoring indoor temperatures. It is easily treated and recognized.

And there are these findings:

¶Knowledge that the immune system declines as we age, alerting doctors to the elderly's diminished ability to fight infection.

¶New research revealing that alcoholism among the elderly is a widespread problem. Alcoholism in the elderly not only debilitates health, it can also mask symptoms of other serious diseases and interfere with the action of critical daily medications. The National Institute of Mental Health, the National Institute on Alcohol Abuse and Alcoholism, the National Institute on Aging, and the Veterans Administration are all studying the problem.

¶A new understanding of the frequency of depression in the elderly and of the host of medical problems it can precipitate.

¶New surgical techniques to treat age-related vision problems: laser surgery for some types of macular degeneration, and
implantable plastic lenses for cataract surgery.

¶Amantadine, rimantadine, and ribavirin — new and better
medications to combat influenza A, a major danger to the elderly.

¶A vaccine against pneumonia.

¶Better control of type II diabetes via home testing and new
diet techniques.

¶A new understanding among the elderly that in order to
thrive in old age, they must consciously form an alliance with the
medical system, and knowledgeably and conscientiously submit to
a steady, continuing stream of diagnostic tests, medical and dental
procedures, and even minor and major surgery. This contract of
care resembles the preventive medical discipline practiced in the
vaccinations and regular checkups of childhood.

Chapter Eight

Decoding and Redesigning Genetic Plans for Future Health

By Philip M. Boffey

Philip M. Boffey covers science and U.S. government science policies for The New York Times.

The young and fast-moving discipline of genetic engineering is raising more hopes and more fears than virtually any other field of medical research. Even before it has conquered a single disease, popular magazines are suggesting that genetic engineering will usher in a golden age, in which the human race will be free from most of the diseases that have ravaged it since the dawn of history. "Imagine a new world, a world in which disease no longer kills or maims," *Parade* magazine, a Sunday newspaper supplement, exulted on January 27, 1985. In that world, the magazine predicted, "all bodily infections, from malaria to viral pneumonia, are eliminated or effectively treated. And every inherited disease, from Down's syndrome (what we commonly call mongolism) to diabetes, is cured in the womb so that the individual is born healthy.

"A science-fiction tale?" the magazine asked rhetorically. "Not at all. We may be well on the way to such a remarkable world because scientists have a new tool — the science of genetic engineering." But offsetting such exuberantly optimistic views of what genetic engineering can accomplish are a host of gloomy warnings from critics, who suggest that genetic engineers, in tampering with human genes that are the very blueprints of life, may bring about a medical, moral, and social catastrophe whose outlines are only dimly perceivable. One Canadian magazine, in apparent seriousness, once suggested that scientists might mix genes from vastly different species together to form "an orange that quacks" or "a flower that can eat you for breakfast." Others fear that scientists will, deliberately or inadvertently, create monstrous new forms of life, perhaps a subhuman class of slaves or a monster like Dr. Frankenstein's. Still others raise the specter of a new eugenics movement — perhaps an attempt to design new genes that would enhance physical and mental capabilities to produce a new "master race."

"Never before in history has such complete power over human life been a possibility," warns Jeremy Rifkin, perhaps the most outspoken lay critic of genetic engineering in the United States. "With the arrival of human genetic engineering, humanity approaches a crossroads in its own political history," he adds. "One day it will be possible to engineer and produce human beings by the same technological design principles as we now employ in our industrial processes." Such a capability, he warns, "presents the human race with the most important political question it has ever had to contend with. Whom do we entrust with the authority to design the blueprints for the future of the human species? Whom do we designate to play God?"

The potentially awesome new powers that may one day be in the hands of scientists led the general secretaries of three major religious bodies — the National Council of Churches, the Synagogue Council of America, and the United States Catholic Conference — to warn the President in 1980 that "We are rapidly moving into a new era of fundamental danger triggered by the rapid growth of genetic engineering. Albeit, there may be opportunity for doing good; the very term suggests the danger."

What is this new technology that evokes such awe and alarm in disparate elements of society? Can it really accomplish as much good, or harm, as people expect? How is this powerful new scientific tool apt to be applied, in the days ahead and in the distant future?

THE TECHNOLOGY

The new science of "genetic engineering" that is exciting such hope and such concern includes a wide range of techniques by which scientists can manipulate the genes that govern the development of all life.

The genes are, by most accounts, the most important of all biological chemicals. They are the chemical blueprints that determine the characteristics of an organism, whether it will grow into a plant, an animal, or a human; its sex, color, blood type, hair, and, in part, its strength and intelligence. Genes control the chemical activity of every cell in the body, specifying what proteins and other substances the cell will produce and what tasks it will perform in the body.

The genes are portions of a long, twisted, complex molecule, known as deoxyribonucleic acid, or DNA, that is found in every human cell, ranging from the cells that make up such organs and structures as the heart, skin, and bones to the sperm and egg cells that pass on genetic traits to the next generation. DNA has been called the master molecule of heredity, and the genes are the various portions of that molecule that govern specific cellular activities and the development of specific human traits. The power to manipulate and rearrange those genes gives biologists more power than they have ever had over human development.

In one sense, genetic engineering has been carried out for thousands of years. For at least 10,000 years, plant and animal breeders have practiced a primitive form of genetic engineering when they use selective breeding to produce organisms with desired characteristics, say a faster racehorse or more ferocious guard dog. Such breeding intermingles the genes of prize animals that have desired characteristics, such as strength or speed, to produce a superior offspring that in turn is used to breed still more superior offspring. Over a span of generations, animals emerge that are different from the original animals, thanks to this crude form of genetic engineering.

But in its modern form, genetic engineering is a very new science, little more than two decades old. Indeed, the term *genetic engineering* was only coined in 1965 to describe new techniques by which scientists could deliberately add specific genetic characteristics directly to cells instead of simply relying on the crude and random process of scrambling genes through breeding.

The most powerful of these new genetic engineering techniques, known as recombinant DNA technology, or gene-splicing, was developed only in the early 1970s. It gave scientists unprecedented power to perform exquisitely precise alterations to the genes. Using this technique, scientists could, for the first time, chemically "snip" out a gene, or portion of the DNA molecule, from one organism and transfer it to another, thus allowing characteristics from the first organism to be engineered into the second organism. By snipping out a gene responsible for, say, an organism's rate of growth, and then reinserting that gene into another organism, the scientists could change the rate of growth of the second organism.

Another powerful technique, known as cell fusion, consists of merging the contents of two cells from different organisms to produce a new hybrid cell that combines their characteristics and continues to reproduce itself. Cell fusion is widely used but is less surgically precise than the gene-splicing techniques of recombinant DNA technology.

By virtually all accounts, genetic engineering is sparking a medical revolution. It has given scientists the power to design better drugs and vaccines by performing genetic manipulations that induce bacteria to produce the new medicines. It has given scientists the opportunity to devise wholly new diagnostic and screening tests for devastating genetic diseases. And, most exciting of all, it offers hope for curing some genetic diseases that have hitherto been deemed hopelessly incurable. On the more distant horizon is the possibility that genetic engineering may eventually give scientists the power to alter the very nature of organisms and the genetic information that these organisms pass on to future generations.

"The recently acquired capability to manipulate the genetic material of all living things is an important — even revolutionary — advance in the trajectory of human knowledge," the President's Commission for the Study of Ethical Problems in Medicine and Biomedical and Behavioral Research commented in 1982.

PHARMACEUTICALS

Genetic engineering has already made its first big contribution to medicine by enabling scientists to manufacture scarce drugs and therapeutic agents in large quantities. They typically do this by inserting a gene that will direct production of the substance into convenient bacteria or yeast cells. The cells, in turn, multiply rapidly and produce millions of identical copies of themselves in a process known as cloning. Each cell in the clone contains the genetic instructions to produce the desired substance, enabling large quantities to be produced under tightly controlled conditions.

The first new genetically engineered agent to gain the approval of American regulatory authorities, in late 1982, was a form of human insulin, a hormone that plays a vital role in enabling the body to convert sugars and other carbohydrates into body fuel. When the body fails to produce enough insulin, the victim develops diabetes, a disease that can cause intense thirst, hunger, weakness, loss of weight, and even coma, with such degenerative changes as arteriosclerosis and cataracts developing in later life.

There is no cure for diabetes, but the disease can be controlled by giving the patient insulin injections that provide enough of the substance to absorb the excess sugars. Traditionally, the insulin has been derived from pigs or cattle because human insulin is not readily available. But now, with the use of recombinant DNA technology, drug companies will be able to produce copious amounts of human insulin.

The development was considered a major scientific achievement, but its practical implications are not immediately clear. Initially, the human insulin was more expensive than animal insulin and showed no clear clinical advantages except in rare cases in which diabetics develop resistance to animal insulin. But if costs can be lowered, or if animal insulin becomes scarcer, the new artificial human insulin will be crucially important.

Other genetically engineered body proteins that are at some stage of research or development include human growth hormones that can be used to promote growth or the healing of fractures; calcium regulators to treat bone disease; reproductive hormones to help infertile couples conceive children; neuroactive peptides that ease pain; and various lymphokines and peptides that help the body's immune defenses fight disease. Genetic engineering is also being used experimentally to produce such blood products as human serum albumin, which is used during surgery to treat shock and burns, and antihemophilic factor, which is used to treat hemophilia, a disorder that prevents blood clotting. Interferon, another substance once thought to be a "wonder drug" against infections of many kinds, is also being made through gene-splicing, thus providing ample quantities for research purposes for the first time.

The greatest immediate promise for genetic engineering probably lies in the production of vaccines and novel antibiotics, according to a 1984 report on commercial biotechnology issued by the Congressional Office of Technology Assessment. The traditional approach to vaccines is to grow a weakened strain of a virus in tissue culture, a tedious chore, and then inoculate people with that strain, with the result that their bodies produce antibodies to protect them against the virus. But with genetic engineering, scientists can produce components of the virus, such as its protein coat, that will stimulate immunity and can be produced in large amounts quickly.

In May 1984, scientists reported the first successful immunizations with a genetically engineered vaccine. They said that an experimental vaccine produced through gene-splicing methods had given healthy adults immunity to hepatitis B virus, the cause of perhaps 200 million cases of liver disease throughout the world. Although an expensive, conventional vaccine against hepatitis B already exists, it is made from material harvested from donated human blood. Thus it is difficult to make, too expensive for worldwide use, and carries some risk of contamination from other substances in the donated human blood. Commercial production of the new vaccine was approved on July 23, 1986, by the Federal Food and Drug Administration, the first such approval for routine human use of any genetically engineered vaccine. Dr. Frank E. Young, the FDA commissioner, called the action "very historic" because similar genetic engineering technologies might soon produce an array of vaccines against such parasitic diseases as malaria, schistosomiasis, and filaria, and such viral diseases as acquired immune deficiency syndrome, or AIDS. "This development opens the door for the production of other vaccines that have so far been impractical, potentially unsafe or impossible to make," he said.

Despite these reported advances, by the mid-1980s some of the initial high expectations for genetic engineering were beginning to fade. Genetic engineering, many entrepreneurs were finding to their dismay, was turning out to be generally more expensive, more time-consuming, and less profitable than originally hoped. The small biotechnology companies that had been formed to exploit the new gene-splicing technologies in the making of pharmaceuticals and other products were universally losing money, and investors were beginning to lose faith in the likelihood of revolutionary advances in the immediate future. "Interest should never have been as high as it was, and it never should have declined so dramatically," said an analyst with Arthur D. Little & Company in Boston, Massachusetts.

Ethicists and doctors were also beginning to raise questions about who should receive the heralded new products and whether the products were wholly beneficial. Genetically engineered human growth hormone, a substance that can be used to treat children of unusually short stature, for example, was at first considered an unqualified blessing. Doctors had previously been forced to rely on human growth hormone harvested from the pituitary glands of corpses, and the readily available supply has generally been limited and expensive. But the abundant quantities of growth hormone that can be produced by genetic engineering are now raising wholly new questions about who should be treated and for what reasons.

Doctors have traditionally used the hormone to treat children who are physiologically deficient in the hormone and would become dwarfs if left untreated. But now that the hormone is likely to become more widely available, ethicists worry that it will be sought out by parents of children who are not particularly short at all, who simply believe that added height will give their children an advantage socially, athletically, or in the business world.

Because even the genetically engineered product is expensive, costing thousands of dollars per year for the course of treatments, ethicists also fret that the new growth hormone may primarily be used by the rich to enhance their social advantages over the poor. By early 1987, scientists were beginning to use growth hormone experimentally to accelerate puberty in cases of delayed adolescence, to help heal wounds and burns, and to treat obesity, the bone loss that occurs in osteoporosis, and the wasting away of muscle that occurs during long periods of bed rest. All of the experiments were in the very early stages and based on unproved theories. As the supplies and potential uses of growth hormone began to mount, so did concerns about possible abuses, ranging from cosmetic applications to a rumored black market among athletes. "There is no question that growth hormone is already being abused in the United States and potentially on a much larger scale in Europe," said Dr. Ron Rosenfeld, associate professor of pediatrics at Stanford University.

None of these worries is peculiar to genetic engineering. But genetic engineering, by making a formerly scarce product more widely available, is raising old ethical questions in new arenas.

GENETIC SCREENING

Medical genetics is finding its first important clinical applications in the areas of screening and diagnosis. Over the past quarter century, scientists have made enormous strides in identifying the genes responsible for certain rare, devastating diseases and in devising tests to identify individuals who carry the defective genes.

Doctors have long sought to counsel individuals who are at

particular risk of giving birth to a deformed child. But for most of this century, such counseling could be done only retrospectively. Only after it had been established that genetic disease had occurred in a family could members of that family be informed of the risks that they, too, might have defective offspring.

Now, however, scientists are developing, and doctors are applying, new screening tests that can detect a few debilitating genetic conditions, and the number and use of such tests is expected to increase dramatically in coming decades.

Over the past three decades, three major forms of genetic screening have been developed. Before birth, prenatal screening is used to determine whether a fetus suffers from a genetic disease. At birth, newborn babies are screened to detect serious genetic diseases that require immediate treatment to avoid health damage or death. And later in life, individuals are sometimes screened to determine whether they have a genetic or chromosomal abnormality that might be harmful to themselves or might cause harm to any offspring they conceive.

The first mass genetic screening in the United States began in the 1960s, when a simple test was developed to detect phenylketonuria, a rare disease in which the lack of an enzyme prevents the body from properly breaking down an amino acid, phenylalanine. Left untreated, the disease generally produces severe mental retardation and physical abnormalities. But once the new test was available, a majority of the states passed laws requiring PKU tests of all newborns. Typically, a drop of blood is taken by pricking the baby's heel, and the level of phenylalanine is measured by laboratory analysis. Those few babies who have too much phenylalanine, a sign of the disease, are immediately put on diets low in phenylalanine to avoid the complications.

Many states also test the baby's blood for other defects and diseases. New York, for example, requires tests for at least seven genetic diseases, including sickle-cell anemia, congenital hyperthyroidism, and five other very rare conditions.

Prenatal screening got started in the mid-1960s when amniocentesis was developed to study the development of the fetus in the uterus. Under this procedure, a needle is inserted through the uterine wall into the amniotic sac that envelops the fetus. Fluids are withdrawn containing cells that have been generated by the fetus. The cells are extracted from the fluid, grown in a culture medium for several weeks, and then studied for abnormalities. The tests are too time-consuming and expensive to be used routinely in mass screening programs, but they are used frequently in certain high-risk cases, for example, to screen women in their thirties who are pregnant for the first time and thus have a higher-than-normal risk of producing defective offspring. During the 1980s, another prenatal diagnostic technique emerged, known as chorionic villus sampling, or CVS, which could detect defects significantly earlier in pregnancy than could amniocentesis, but with greater risk to the fetus. In this procedure, a plastic tube is inserted up through the vagina into the uterus. Suction is applied to withdraw tissue samples from the outside of the fetal gestational sac, and these samples are then analyzed in the laboratory for chromosomal and genetic defects. By mid-1986, an estimated 10,000 CVS procedures had been performed in Europe and the United States. In skilled hands, the CVS procedure appeared twice as risky as amniocentesis, causing loss of the fetus in perhaps 1 percent of the cases. But the great advantage of CVS was that it could provide results in the first trimester of pregnancy, when abortion is relatively easy, whereas amniocentesis was not effective until the second trimester, when abortion is a major procedure.

Prenatal diagnostic tests have been proliferating rapidly. At least 190 genetically related metabolic defects and congenital disorders can now be diagnosed before birth, as can many defects in the chromosomal structure that houses the genes.

The first large-scale genetic screening program for adult carriers of a disease started in 1970 with a pilot program to detect carriers of Tay-Sachs disease in the Jewish population. The victims of Tay-Sachs disease are children who inherit a gene that fails to function properly, with the result that the body does not produce enough of an enzyme needed to break down fatty substances in the brain. The accumulation of these substances disrupts the brain; the children regress into a vegetative state and almost always die within two to four years.

There is no known cure. But if adults who have a gene for

Tay-Sachs can be identified, they can be counseled that, if they mate with another adult carrying the gene, there is a 25 percent risk that their offspring will come down with the disease. It is also possible to determine by prenatal blood testing whether a fetus still in the womb is suffering from Tay-Sachs, making it possible for parents to decide whether they want to abort the doomed fetus or go through with the birth and face a lingering and painful death for the child.

By 1981, some 350,000 young Jewish adults had been screened for Tay-Sachs throughout the world, and 337 carrier-couples, a tiny percentage of the whole, had been detected among them. The number of children born with Tay-Sachs disease in North America, which had risen toward 100 in some years before 1970, dropped to little more than a dozen by 1980. By most accounts, Tay-Sachs screening had been an enormous success.

Tests were also developed during the 1970s to detect the genetic defects that can lead to sickle-cell anemia and beta-thalassemia, two diseases that affect the oxygen-carrying capacity of the blood. By 1986, the ability to screen for faulty genes appeared to be reducing substantially the amount of some genetic disorders in the population. Dr. Haig H. Kazazian, Jr., of the Johns Hopkins Medical Institutions in Baltimore, estimated that the number of new cases of beta-thalassemia had dropped by 50 percent or more in recent years in some parts of the country and some parts of the Mediterranean basin where the disease is common. He predicted that the tests would have a similar effect on hemophilia and Duchenne muscular dystrophy in the next few years.

In recent years, scientists have also found a genetic finger-print that appears to identify at least some carriers of the gene for Huntington's disease, a progressive deterioration of brain cells that leads to writhing and twisting, depression, dementia, and death in middle age.

Eventually, doctors expect to be able to detect a person's susceptibility to a wide range of other diseases. Already, they have found genetic abnormalities that affect the body's ability to handle fats, one of the risk factors for heart attacks in the middle-aged and elderly. They have also found genes that affect the immune system and that may be involved in Alzheimer's disease, a common form of progressive mental deterioration. And they hope, eventually, to identify genes that predispose people to cancer, diabetes, and mental illness. In May 1986, medical researchers reported the first successful use of genetic-probe technology to predict the likelihood that a child would develop cancer. The scientists were able to tell four sets of parents whether or not their infants carried genes that predisposed them to retinoblastoma, a form of eye cancer, and in each case their predictions proved right. In February 1987, separate groups of scientists reported strong evidence that a defective gene causes the hereditary form of Alzheimer's disease and the first evidence that a defective gene, or possibly multiple genes, predispose their bearers to manic depression, a major form of mental illness.

Genetic screening has thus far been used on a limited basis, to test newborns for a few rare diseases or to screen selected population groups, such as Jews or blacks, for specific genetic conditions that afflict them more often than the general population. But the era of mass screening appears to be drawing near. In 1983, a presidential commission, called the President's Commission for the Study of Ethical Problems in Medicine and Biomedical and Behavioral Research, said there is likely to be a "huge demand" for genetic screening tests to determine whether parents are likely to have defective offspring. It predicted that a screening test for the most prevalent lethal inherited disease, cystic fibrosis, would be in hand by the end of the 1980s, thus making possible "a new program of mass genetic screening of vast proportions." Cystic fibrosis afflicts about one in every 1,800 newborns, damaging the lungs and digestive system and generally killing its victims before the age of twenty. Depending on scientific advances, various screening tests might be used on prospective parents, pregnant women, or newborn infants.

"Genetics is only beginning to play a significant part in health care," the commission said. "Before the end of the century, however, genetic screening and counseling are certain to become major components in both public health and individual medical care." The time "can already be envisioned," it added, when virtually all information about a person's "abnormal" genes and chromosomes will be readily accessible.

The prospect of increased genetic screening is already raising serious ethical concerns. It will almost certainly be possible to detect many genetic defects in the fetus before doctors have the ability to correct the genetic problem. This will undoubtedly lead to an increase in abortions to avoid a genetically diseased child, a prospect that horrifies many antiabortion groups in the United States.

Genetic screening is also being considered by many corporations as a tool to screen workers for signs of genetic defects that might make them especially vulnerable to toxic chemicals. That prospect has raised concerns that workers so identified might be stigmatized as defective. It also raises fears that employers might act unjustly on the basis of the information, that they might exclude workers from certain jobs because of their genetic vulnerabilities and fail to provide them with a comparable job.

"The fundamental basis of our egalitarian attitudes toward individuals could erode," warns Representative John Dingell, chairman of a House committee with jurisdiction over biotechnology. "As we describe fully the genetic makeup of an individual, we could become less and less likely to treat everyone as having equal potential and deserving equal opportunities."

The presidential ethics commission warned that genetic screening raises "important ethical and legal concerns" about who should have access to the tests and the information they reveal, whether the tests should be voluntary or compulsory, and what they should be used for. It threw its moral weight against using amniocentesis to determine the sex of a fetus so that parents could abort a fetus of unwanted sex. It also opposed mandatory screening in an effort to produce a "genetically healthy society" or other "vague and politically abusable social ideals."

GENE THERAPY

Of all the potential applications of genetic engineering, none excites such enthusiasm, and such dread, as gene therapy, the use of the new genetic techniques to modify the human genes so as to cure disease, or even change the course of human development.

Thus far, there are no cures for genetic disease. The only treatments available once a genetic defect is diagnosed in a patient are palliative, aimed at modifying the consequences of a defective gene rather than repairing the defect. Thus, parents carrying defective genes can avoid passing them on to their children either by abstaining from having children or by aborting a fetus that is genetically impaired. Similarly, children who lack some crucial body substance because of a genetic defect can be supplied with that substance artificially, as youngsters who lack sufficient growth hormone are now treated with hormone injections.

But there is not yet any "cure" for a genetic disease. There is no effective gene therapy to replace a harmful gene or to activate an inactive one. The search for such cures is currently the leading edge of medical genetics.

Genetic diseases cause a significant burden of human suffering. There are 2,000 to 3,000 known genetic diseases whose roots can be traced to specific genes or to known inheritance patterns. Prominent disorders such as sickle-cell anemia, hemophilia, cystic fibrosis, Huntington's disease, Duchenne muscular dystrophy, and many others are caused by defects in a single gene. These diseases are individually rare but collectively they cause an immense amount of human suffering. As many as 2 percent of all newborn infants suffer from such single-gene disorders. And countless other individuals suffer from more complex diseases that may be importantly influenced by the genes. Cancer, the second leading killer disease in the United States, is believed to be caused, in large part, by genetic alterations in the oncogenes. And heart disease, the leading killer of Americans, may have an important genetic component.

Eventually, gene therapy may be applied to a wide variety of these diseases and may employ any of several different approaches. But the first human gene therapy will almost certainly use the simplest technology and be directed at a simple disorder caused by a defect in a single gene.

It will also be applied, initially, only to somatic cells, the kind that compose most of the body's tissues and affect only the individual patient. Gene therapy of the germ cells, such as the sperm or egg cells that pass characteristics on to subsequent generations, is still a long way off. Such germ-cell gene therapy is far more difficult to perform, and it raises ethical issues that are not present in somatic-cell therapy.

The simplest form of gene therapy is gene insertion, in which a normally functioning gene is added to a cell in which a defective gene is present. As a result, two opposing chemical processes take place in the cell. The old gene continues to produce its defective product, while the new gene begins to produce the normal product. The normal product, in many cases, is expected to be enough to alleviate the symptoms of disease.

More complicated forms of gene therapy will include gene modification, in which a defective gene already in place is altered, and gene surgery, in which a defective gene is excised and replaced with its normal counterpart. Such complicated manipulations have already been performed in some viruses, yeast, and bacteria, but they are not yet ready for application to animals or humans.

In a crude sense, the era of gene therapy started years ago, with two unsuccessful attempts abroad to implant new genes in human beings. In the early 1970s, doctors used a primitive form of gene therapy — not involving recombinant DNA techniques — to treat three German sisters suffering from a rare genetic disease that caused them to develop a high level of a substance called arginine in their blood, a condition that leads to severe mental retardation. The doctors deliberately infected the sisters with a virus that they hoped would transfer a gene enabling the sisters to convert the arginine into safer substances. However, the treatment was unsuccessful, and the buildup of arginine continued.

In 1980, Dr. Martin Cline, a physician at the University of California at Los Angeles, created an uproar in the scientific community when he became the first to apply recombinant DNA techniques to the treatment of human disease in two experiments that most scientists considered rash and premature. Dr. Cline attempted to transplant genes into two young women in Italy and Israel who were suffering from beta-thalassemia, an inherited blood disorder caused by a defective gene for beta globin, one of the building blocks for hemoglobin, the oxygen-carrying molecule in the blood. Dr. Cline withdrew samples of bone marrow from each of the patients, mixed them with normal hemoglobin genes, and restored the treated bone marrow cells into the patients, hoping that the corrected cells would find a niche in bone cavities and multiply. The attempt failed; it neither helped nor harmed the patients. But Dr. Cline was stripped of his grants and resigned from his post as chairman of a university division because he had rushed ahead without appropriate animal work or the permission of ethical review boards.

The dispute over Dr. Cline's experiments probably slowed the rush toward gene therapy, but in 1987 American doctors were again preparing for experiments to insert new genes into an appropriate patient, and the first such experiment in the United States was expected to take place within a year or two.

The key factor making such experiments possible is a new method for inserting foreign genes into human cells that is far more effective than the method used by Dr. Cline. Special genetically engineered viruses, known as retroviruses, are used to infect a cell, carrying with them the new genes to be inserted and spliced into the cell's own genetic material. Scientists are also working on other insertion techniques, including fusing two cells together, injecting the new genes through tiny needles, and various chemical and physical treatments to encourage cells to absorb new genetic materials.

The most likely candidates for the initial American experiment in gene therapy are three serious, often lethal, extremely rare diseases for which no treatment now exists. One is ADA enzyme deficiency, a disorder in which a defective gene results in lack of an enzyme known as adenosine deaminase, leading to an accumulation of toxic chemicals in the body that destroys the immune defenses. Another contender is PNP enzyme deficiency, in which another defective gene results in a similar accumulation of toxic chemicals and harm to the body's defenses. In both diseases, simple childhood ailments, such as diaper rash, can lead to serious illness and even death.

The treatment for these diseases will involve removing defective cells from the body, genetically altering them in the laboratory, and then restoring them to the body. By performing the key alterations outside the body, there is little chance of affecting either the germ cells or any other body tissues that need not be treated.

The experiments are expected to have a wide tolerance for error. Doctors believe that if the new genes they insert produce some of the needed enzymes, even if substantially fewer than normal, the treatment will still benefit the patient. And should the new genes overproduce the needed enzymes, the results would still be much less harmful to the patients than if they were left untreated, doctors reason.

Another early contender for gene therapy is Lesch-Nyhan syndrome, a rare inherited disorder in which a defective gene results in lack of an essential enzyme. As a result, uric acid builds up, causing gout and severe kidney damage. By unknown processes, the disease also affects the brain, producing uncontrollable urges to spit, curse, bite off the fingers and lips, and bang the head against walls. If this disease is treated by gene therapy, doctors would remove white blood cells from the bone marrow of a Lesch-Nyhan patient, use a retrovirus to insert new genes into the cells in the laboratory, thus causing them to produce the missing enzyme, and then reinsert the cells in the patient. The chief worry is that the bone marrow treatments will cure only some of the biochemical defects in the patient but will not eliminate the brain effects of the disease. Although some exuberant scientists had once predicted that the first clinical attempt at human gene therapy would take place in 1985, the task proved more difficult than expected, partly because retroviral vectors were hard to design well and partly because genes that were inserted into a defective cell did not always cure it. Expert projections of the arrival of gene therapy became decidedly more cautious in 1986 and 1987. At the annual meeting of the Institute of Medicine, part of the prestigious National Academy of Sciences, in October 1986, experts agreed that ADA deficiency was likely to be the first target for gene therapy. But David W. Martin, Jr., vice-president for research at Genentech, Inc., a leading biotechnology company based in San Francisco, noted that his group had only achieved "adequate ADA expression" in cells treated in a laboratory dish, not in whole mice or primates, indicating that there was "a long way to go." Dr. Leon Rosenberg, chairman of the meeting and dean of the medical school at Yale University, concluded that "We stand close to attempting to cure certain very rare and very serious human genetic disorders using gene therapy" but that "significant hurdles still remain," indicating that "gene therapy, while near at hand, is not in the immediate offing."

Whatever disease is ultimately targeted, the treatments are not expected to raise unusual ethical problems or unusual risks, according to most religious, ethical, and medical thinkers. Senator Albert Gore, Jr., Democrat of Tennessee, who held hearings on genetic engineering while a member of the House of Representatives, reported that a strong consensus had emerged on the acceptability of somatic-cell therapy to help individual patients.

Similarly, the Congressional Office of Technology Assessment, in a 1984 background paper on human gene therapy, stated: "Gene therapy in humans will first be done in cells from an organ or tissue other than germ cells. Therefore, because cells that are used in reproduction are not involved, gene therapy of this type is quite similar to other kinds of medical therapy, and does not pose new kinds of risks.

"When considering gene therapy that does not result in inherited change," the paper added, "the factor that most distinguishes it from other medical technologies is its conspicuousness in the public eye; otherwise it can be viewed as simply another tool to help individuals overcome an illness."

The major question is when to begin clinical trials of somatic-cell gene therapy, not whether to begin them at all, the OTA paper said.

The diseases for which somatic-cell gene therapy is now contemplated are quite rare. Only forty to fifty patients in the entire world are reported to have ADA deficiency, and only nine patients have the even rarer PNP deficiency. About 200 cases of the slightly more common Lesch-Nyhan syndrome occur in the United States each year. Even so, the total number of patients suffering from the five diseases most likely to be the first candidates for gene therapy is probably less than 300 a year in the United States, according to the Office of Technology Assessment.

If gene therapy is used only sparingly in the near future, as these numbers suggest, then the social impact of gene therapy will be less than that of many other medical practices.

The most troubling potential application of gene therapy is germ-cell modification that could cause changes transmissible to the patient's children and on to succeeding generations. There is bound to be pressure for such germ-cell changes because, if doctors can cure a simple genetic defect in adult somatic cells, why not cure the defect in the germ cells as well to save future offspring from needless suffering?

The male sperm cells may be difficult to alter genetically because they are small and difficult to penetrate, and would have to be treated in vast numbers. But the larger and more easily manipulated female egg cells might well be altered after they are extruded from the ovary and before fertilization. Alternatively, fertilized embryos at a very early stage of development might be the target for genetic manipulation. In that case, embryos that carry abnormal genes might be removed from the woman, genetically altered in the laboratory, and returned to the female for further development. Every cell in the young embryo would presumably have been altered, including its germ cells.

Few critics dispute the desirability of eliminating genetic disease. But once doctors start tampering with the germ cells, some critics fear, the way is open for questionable manipulation of human characteristics to produce more perfect human beings.

"Once we decide to begin the process of human genetic engineering, there is really no logical place to stop," warns Jeremy Rifkin. "If diabetes, sickle-cell anemia, and cancer are to be cured by altering the genetic makeup of an individual, why not proceed to other 'disorders': myopia, color blindness, lefthandedness? Indeed, what is to preclude a society from deciding that a certain skin color is a disorder?"

In 1983, fifty-six religious leaders and eight scientists and ethicists joined Mr. Rifkin in a resolution calling for a ban on germ-line experiments. "The redesign of the human species by genetic engineering technology irreversibly alters the composition of the human gene pool for all future generations of human life," the resolution said. Such technical advances will require that "decisions be made as to which genetic traits should be programmed into the human gene pool and which should be eliminated," the resolution added. "No individual, group of individuals, or institutions can legitimately claim the right or authority to make such decisions on behalf of the rest of the species."

But warnings such as these carry little weight with most patients suffering from a devastating genetic disease. Ola Huntley, the mother of three children with sickle-cell anemia, has argued strenuously in favor of gene therapy. "I resent the fact that a few well-meaning individuals have presented arguments strong enough to curtail the scientific technology which promises to give some hope to those suffering from a genetic disease," she said. "Aren't those theologians and politicians playing God? Aren't they deciding what's best for me without any knowledge of my suffering? I am very angry that anyone would presume to deny my children and my family the essential genetic treatment of a genetic disease."

Whether germ-line gene therapy will ever become important is not yet clear. The OTA paper suggests that gene therapies to change inherited characteristics "are unlikely to be undertaken in humans in the near future because they are technically too difficult, are perceived as ethically problematic, and may not prove superior to existing technologies." The paper concludes, for example, that gene therapy on early embryos is unlikely because there is no safe and effective test to determine whether an embryo is normal or not. If there were such a test, many experts say, it would almost certainly be used to select a normal embryo that would then be allowed to follow the natural course of development. There would be little point in using gene therapy on an abnormal embryo, with all the uncertainties and risks that such therapy would entail.

Scientists are at the very beginning of the revolution in genetic engineering. They have yet to cure even the simplest kind of genetic diseases, those caused by a defect in a single gene. Far more difficult are diseases that involve the interaction of many genes or disruption of the chromosomal structures that house the genes. And scientists are a very long way from being able to improve such complex traits as intelligence and physical stamina that are determined by the interactions of many genes with each other, with their products, and with the environment.

Genetic engineering has given scientists a powerful new tool to investigate and manipulate the fundamental machinery of life. The technology is developing quickly, and on many fronts. But the most troublesome potential applications lie far enough off in the future to permit reasoned study of their implications well in advance of their arrival. The time to start such study, most experts say, is now.